IAMSE Manuals

Editor-in-Chief

Emine Ercikan Abali, CUNY School of Medicine, New York, USA

Editorial Board

Femmie de Vegt, Department of Health Evidence, Radboud University Medical Centre, Nijmegen, The Netherlands

Robin Ann Harvan, School of Arts and Sciences, MCPHS University, Boston, USA

Sarah Lerchenfeldt, Rochester, USA

Mary Mathews, Kasturba Medical College, Manipal, Karnataka, India

Carolina Restini, Michigan State University, Clinton Township, USA

Douglas Spicer, Biddeford Campus, University of New England, Biddeford, USA

The book series IAMSE Manuals is established to rapidly deploy the latest developments and best evidence-based examples in medical education, offering all who teach in healthcare the most current information to succeed in their task by publishing short "how-to-guides" on a variety of topics relevant to medical teaching. The series aims to make the best and latest evidence-based methods for teaching in medical education to educators around the world, to improve the quality of teaching in healthcare education, and to establish greater interest in the teaching of the medical sciences.

David L. Kok • David Seignior
Michelle Barrett
Editors

Best Practices in Online Education

A Guide for Health Professional Educators

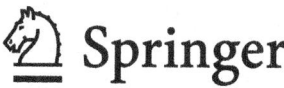

Editors
David L. Kok
Peter MacCallum Cancer Centre/University
of Melbourne
Melbourne, VIC, Australia

David Seignior
University of Melbourne
Melbourne, VIC, Australia

Michelle Barrett
Victorian Comprehensive Cancer Centre
Melbourne, VIC, Australia

ISSN 2673-9291　　　　　　　ISSN 2673-9305　(electronic)
IAMSE Manuals
ISBN 978-3-031-90348-9　　　ISBN 978-3-031-90349-6　(eBook)
https://doi.org/10.1007/978-3-031-90349-6

© International Association of Medical Science Educators 2025

This work is subject to copyright. All rights are solely and exclusively licensed by the Publisher, whether the whole or part of the material is concerned, specifically the rights of translation, reprinting, reuse of illustrations, recitation, broadcasting, reproduction on microfilms or in any other physical way, and transmission or information storage and retrieval, electronic adaptation, computer software, or by similar or dissimilar methodology now known or hereafter developed.
The use of general descriptive names, registered names, trademarks, service marks, etc. in this publication does not imply, even in the absence of a specific statement, that such names are exempt from the relevant protective laws and regulations and therefore free for general use.
The publisher, the authors and the editors are safe to assume that the advice and information in this book are believed to be true and accurate at the date of publication. Neither the publisher nor the authors or the editors give a warranty, expressed or implied, with respect to the material contained herein or for any errors or omissions that may have been made. The publisher remains neutral with regard to jurisdictional claims in published maps and institutional affiliations.

This Springer imprint is published by the registered company Springer Nature Switzerland AG.
The registered company address is: Gewerbestrasse 11, 6330 Cham, Switzerland

If disposing of this product, please recycle the paper.

Preface

There has been extensive growth in the utilisation and availability of online health professional education in recent years. This has been driven by a combination of factors including rapid advances in the capability of educational technology, increasing use of digital technology for learning and work, COVID-19, and worsening time pressures on clinical learners driving them towards more flexible approaches to access education.

In line with this, educational research into the pedagogical underpinnings of online education has also significantly advanced. However, given the speed of these developments (and the number of competing priorities for health professional educators' attention), many educators remain unfamiliar with online educational techniques, their best practice pedagogy, and the practicalities of designing and delivering these learning experiences.

As the team behind an extensive portfolio of online health professional education programming, we experienced first-hand the challenge of finding quality guidance and references. After overcoming these obstacles and achieving some level of success with our programs, we began receiving frequent requests from colleagues for advice and seminars on our expertise and insights. Thus, it seemed like the obvious next step to compile and curate our knowledge and resources into a single, handy reference manual for working health professional educators to refer to when incorporating online techniques into their own curricula. As such, we set about writing this manual.

In this manual, we aim to quickly bring educators up to speed on the key considerations, capabilities, pedagogical underpinnings and implementation frameworks necessary for online education. This is like saying we provide the bricks, tools and engineering principles that you need to build a house. In addition, we provide a series of useful 'tips and tricks' for each stage that should help to fast-track your construction process. What we do not do, however, is describe what you should build or what it should look like. Do you want to build a 40-storey, skyline-defining tower or a sound 2-bedroom cottage? That's up to you. This is the challenge of any text which tackles curriculum design—being too prescriptive constrains and limits the final output and risks producing repetitive 'cookie-cutter' experiences, when educational curricula can (and should) be of all shapes, sizes and designs.

Therefore, we acknowledge this book is not the *final* word on all things online learning. But conversely, we hope that it will be the *first* book reached for when commencing an online curriculum build. Thus, providing a gateway for innovative, passionate health professional educators worldwide to begin their personal and organisational online education evolutions.

Melbourne, VIC, Australia	David L. Kok
Melbourne, VIC, Australia	David Seignior
Melbourne, VIC, Australia	Michelle Barrett

Contents

1 **Online Health Professional Education: Core Educational Theories, Opportunities and Challenges** 1
David L. Kok, Michelle Barrett, David Bowser, Alicia Mew, Sathana Dushyanthen, and David Seignior

2 **Designing Effective, Online Health Professional Curricula** 29
David L. Kok, Michelle Barrett, Sathana Dushyanthen, and David Seignior

3 **Contexts and Conditions for Online Learning Success** 57
Michelle Barrett, David Seignior, and Alicia Mew

4 **Best Practice Design and Delivery with Digital Learning Tools** 75
Sathana Dushyanthen, David L. Kok, Alicia Mew, and Michelle Barrett

5 **Teaching and Facilitating Online** 113
Alicia Mew, Bhaumik Shah, and David L. Kok

6 **Multidisciplinary, Interdisciplinary and Interprofessional Online Education** 133
David Seignior, Michelle Barrett, and David L. Kok

7 **Applications of Artificial Intelligence to Health Professional Education** 163
Thomas Cochrane, David Seignior, and David L. Kok

8 **Implementing and Leading Online Education Transformation** 185
David Bowser

About the Editors and Contributors

About the Editors

David Kok is an Oncologist and award-winning Medical Educator dually employed by the Peter MacCallum Cancer Centre and The University of Melbourne. He is currently the Chair of the Cancer Education and Training Advisory Committee for the Victorian Comprehensive Cancer Alliance, Head of Campus at Peter MacCallum Cancer Centre Moorabbin and Chief of Training for the Royal Australian and New Zealand College of Radiology's Faculty of Radiation Oncology. His expertise is in designing and delivering tailored education experiences for clinical learners. He has led the development of numerous courses incorporating interactive case scenarios, fully animated videos and virtual reality simulations. David sits on a range of national and international educational committees and has published and lectured widely relating to best practice in tertiary and postgraduate health professional education.

David Seignior is a multidisciplinary teacher and researcher in the Faculty of Education, at the University of Melbourne. Prior to this, he was a senior learning designer with the Melbourne School of Professional and Continuing Education (MSPACE), where his main focus was on health professional education. His learning design experience includes with the University of Melbourne and Victorian Comprehensive Cancer Centre (VCCC) Alliance's wholly online Master of Cancer Sciences course. David now teaches and researches in philosophy of education, environmental education and climate change, and diversity and inclusion in teacher training and practice. His doctorate was a phenomenological inquiry into the experiences of students undertaking wholly online interprofessional education in cancer sciences.

Michelle Barrett has worked in health professional education since 2001, predominantly in curriculum writing and educational development and delivery in the medical undergraduate, postgraduate, specialist and professional education and training arena. Her special interests focus on transformative learning practice, program evaluation, consumers as educators and innovative educational technology. Since 2018, she has been the Head of Education and Training at the Victorian Comprehensive Cancer Centre Alliance, where she develops, curates and manages educational programming that supports knowledge and skill development for the clinical and research cancer workforce. Prior to that, she was the Manager of Professional Development at the Royal Australasian College of Surgeons, Manager of Curriculum and Training Development at the Royal Australasian College of Medical Administrators and Lecturer, Centre for Medical and Health Sciences Education at Monash University. Michelle has an honours qualification in science, postgraduate qualification in scientific communications and Master of Professional Education and Training.

About the Authors

David Bowser PhD (Neuroscience), MBA, is the CEO and Founder of Curio. He specialises in education R&D and strategy consulting and was involved in producing educational models and business strategies for universities, as well as leading the creation of Curio's online education services.

Thomas Cochrane BE, BD, GDHE, MTS, MComp (Hons), PhD (Monash), SCMALT, is an Associate Professor Technology Enhanced Learning in Higher Education at the Centre for the Study of Higher Education, the University of Melbourne. They specialise in mobile learning, immersive reality and the impact of artificial intelligence in higher education and have worked alongside health professional educators in Paramedicine, Physiotherapy, Nursing, Anatomy and Physiology.

Sathana Dushyanthen BSc, MSc, PhD, GradCertUniTeach is an Educator and Researcher at the University of Melbourne (UoM). She co-led the development of the Master of Cancer Sciences program and now works in the Centre for Digital Transformations of Health as an Academic Specialist. As a Learning Scientist, she specialises in the use of new and engaging technologies in Medical Education such as gamification, virtual/augmented reality, graphics, interaction and animation, to enhance engagement online.

Alicia Mew BTeach, Barts, GradCert eLearning, MEd (eLearning), is an E-learning Developer at the Victorian Comprehensive Cancer Centre (VCCC) Alliance and is an adult and primary educator who specialises in the development and facilitation of eLearning, blended and face-to-face course design. Her passion for education is to promote and invest in learning that thinks beyond the traditional, strengthens learners' capabilities and strives to be transformational.

Bhaumik Shah MBBS, MD, FRACP, GradCertClinEd, is a medical oncologist and educator at the University of Melbourne. They specialise in clinical education at undergraduate, postgraduate and interdisciplinary levels for oncology. They coordinate multiple subjects in the University's Master of Cancer Sciences program.

List of Figures

Fig. 1.1	Three-stage model of human memory - From Kok et al. [76]	17
Fig. 1.2	Multimedia Learning Theory. Multimedia learning is an active process consisting of a combination of words and images that are interpreted via sensory memory. It is processed by two channels (auditory and visual), which have finite capacity but can be used simultaneously. The working memory organises these sounds and images and integrates them together with prior knowledge from long-term memory; this is then encoded into long-term memory (adapted from Krumm et al. [82])	19
Fig. 2.1	The Technological, Pedagogical, Content Knowledge (TPACK) framework (from Koehler and Mishra [16]) (Reproduced by permission of the publisher, © 2012 by tpack.org)	34
Fig. 2.2	Kern's curriculum development model with tips for educators (from Kok et al. [25])	37
Fig. 2.3	Educational Leadership skills required in online education	42
Fig. 2.4	Online teaching and facilitation skills required in online education	42
Fig. 2.5	Instructional Design skills required in online education	43
Fig. 2.6	Content Creation skills required in online education	43
Fig. 2.7	Educational technology and video production skills required in online education	44
Fig. 2.8	Evaluation and education research skills required in online education	44
Fig. 2.9	Example of a subject roadmap for a cancer science subject	46
Fig. 2.10	Digital platform administration skills required in online education	51
Fig. 2.11	Event support skills required in online education	51
Fig. 3.1	The contextual 'building blocks' that influence online learning	60
Fig. 3.2	Supportive practices for aligning instructional design with online learning	61
Fig. 3.3	Supportive practices for aligning social interactions with online learning	62

Fig. 3.4	Supportive practices for aligning organisational culture with online learning	63
Fig. 3.5	Supportive practices for aligning organisational structures with online learning	64
Fig. 3.6	Supportive practices for aligning learner demographics with online learning	65
Fig. 3.7	Supportive practices for aligning learner motivators and drivers with online learning	66
Fig. 3.8	Supportive practices for aligning societal constructs with online learning	67
Fig. 3.9	Supportive practices for aligning physical and virtual spaces with online learning	68
Fig. 4.1	Examples of the types of videos that can be created outside of PowerPoint slides with voiceover. (**a**) Presenter with a touch screen where you can point and highlight different aspects. (**b**) *In situ* demonstrations of procedures with voice-over and annotation. (**c**) Simulated multidisciplinary meeting, round table discussion of real-world patient cases from different perspectives. (**d**) Expert interviews or expert panel with various perspectives represented on a current debate or hot topic	79
Fig. 4.2	Examples of different types of animations that can be used in HPE. (**a**) 2D molecular signalling processes. (**b**) 3D cellular processes, (**c**) 2D character depictions of clinical scenarios. (**d**) 2D doodle drawing of medical processes. (Stills are taken from videos produced by our team and are also available on Science in Motion and YouTube.)	83
Fig. 4.3	Examples of (**a**) graphics [17] and (**b**) infographics that can be used in HPE [18]. (**a**) example of an interactive graphic that demonstrates the population attributable fraction (PAF) and data on cancer incidence by cancer site and infectious agent. It contains clickable elements and circles are proportional. (**b**) Represents a static infographic that presents information and statistics for after-hours care options	86
Fig. 4.4	Tips, steps and multimedia principles for designing visuals for text or video [18]	88
Fig. 4.5	Examples of (**a**) augmented reality and (**b**) virtual reality in HPE. (**a**) The AR app 'HoloHuman' displays a virtual cadaver, projected on a real-world space. The learner can interact with the model and user interface through the use of a HoloLens headset. Structures, organs and systems can be examined, supported by visual narratives and digital dissection tools (3D4 Medical from Elsevier, 2020) [31]. (**b**) Fully immersive VR environment exploring communication skills between patients and clinicians [32]. Reproduced under CC BY 4.0	94

Fig. 4.6	Medical influencers on TikTok for the #MedEd hashtag. (**a**) Dr Todorovic explaining the role of a hormone using whiteboard illustration. (**b**) Dr Mike discussing the polycystic ovarian syndrome symptoms. (**c**) Dr Leslie discussing the criteria for the COVID-19 booster vaccination	106
Fig. 5.1	Depth of Change	115
Fig. 5.2	The Community of Inquiry Framework	116
Fig. 5.3	Roles and Responsibilities of the Online Educator	117
Fig. 5.4	Mezirow's 10 phases of transformative learning linked to Andragogy [11, 15, 16]	121
Fig. 5.5	Communities of Practice and Transformative Learning	125
Fig. 6.1	Multidisciplinary or multiprofessional education	136
Fig. 6.2	Interdisciplinary or interprofessional education	137
Fig. 6.3	Community of Inquiry	138
Fig. 6.4	Constructive alignment	145
Fig. 6.5	Kirkpatrick's typology of educational outcomes	146
Fig. 6.6	Amended Miller's pyramid	147
Fig. 6.7	Nested structure of the Master of Cancer Sciences (Case study 1). Source [39]	158
Fig. 6.8	Learning Health Systems (Case study 2). Source [41]	159

List of Tables

Table 1.1	Timeline of major HPE advances	4
Table 1.2	Online learning pedagogical domains – adapted from Means et al. [29] and Hodges et al. [30]	6
Table 1.3	Summary of learning theories relevant to online education and their design implications	15
Table 2.1	Example of how pedagogical strategies were mapped to address the specific needs of cancer professionals in an online degree in cancer sciences (Excerpt from Lai Kwon et al. [29])	40
Table 2.2	Example of using Kern's Six-Step Approach in the Design of the University of Melbourne Master of Cancer Science Curriculum (From Lai Kwon et al. [29])	49
Table 4.1	Evidence-based multimedia learning principles (adapted from Yue et al. [13] and Mayer [14])	81
Table 4.2	Social learning platforms commonly used in higher education, along with their descriptions	90
Table 4.3	Simulation principles (adapted from Lopreiato and Sawyer [33])	96
Table 4.4	Principles for scenario or game design (adapted from Argueta-Munoz et al. [44])	103
Table 4.5	Design principles for creating TikTok videos (adapted from Lacey [52])	105
Table 5.1	Roles and Common Tasks of the Online Educator	118
Table 5.2	Important Factors to Define Context of Online Education	123
Table 5.3	Key mechanisms to support online educators	127
Table 8.1	Example of a transformation roadmap	191
Table 8.2	Risk Evaluation Matrix	196
Table 8.3	Mitigation Strategies	197
Table 8.4	Monitoring and Reporting	197

Chapter 1
Online Health Professional Education: Core Educational Theories, Opportunities and Challenges

David L. Kok, Michelle Barrett, David Bowser, Alicia Mew, Sathana Dushyanthen, and David Seignior

Abstract Online Education is well suited to health professional education (HPE) due to a combination of features including flexibility, accessibility, yield, and personalisation ability. As such, there is a growing appetite for health professional education programs to be delivered either in part, or in full, via online methods.

Our understanding of the pedagogical underpinnings of digital learning tools and techniques has rapidly advanced in recent years, significantly accelerated by COVID-19. However, given the recency and speed of these academic developments, many health professional educators remain unfamiliar with the nuances of the tools and techniques, their evidence base, and the practicalities of designing and delivering these learning experiences in a best-practice manner.

This introductory chapter begins by examining the definition and ways of classifying online education. It then outlines the potential opportunities for health professional educators who embrace online learning and balances this against some of the challenges of online education. It concludes by summarising the key educational learning theories that can be leveraged in online learning and thus result in more effective learning experiences.

D. L. Kok (✉)
Peter MacCallum Cancer Centre, Melbourne, VIC, Australia

University of Melbourne, Melbourne, VIC, Australia

Monash University, Melbourne, VIC, Australia
e-mail: dkok@unimelb.edu.au; dkok@unimelb.edu.au

M. Barrett · A. Mew
Victorian Comprehensive Cancer Centre, Melbourne, VIC, Australia

D. Bowser
Curio Group, Melbourne, VIC, Australia

S. Dushyanthen · D. Seignior
University of Melbourne, Melbourne, VIC, Australia

© The Author(s), under exclusive license to Springer Nature Switzerland AG 2025
D. L. Kok et al. (eds.), *Best Practices in Online Education*, IAMSE Manuals, https://doi.org/10.1007/978-3-031-90349-6_1

Key Points

- Online Education is well suited to HPE because of its flexibility, accessibility, yield, and personalisation ability.
- Effective online education design should take into account the strengths and weaknesses of the online medium.
- Understanding and applying core educational theories will result in more effective online learning experiences.
- Online education is a natural evolution of educational science, and all educators should be proficient at it.

1.1 Introduction

Health professional education (HPE) (Also commonly known as Health Profession Education or Health Professions Education) is the crucial means by which the healthcare workforce is created, maintained and upskilled. In doing this, it is subject to a unique set of external pressures.

Clinical knowledge is rapidly evolving, driven by a thriving medical research sphere [1, 2]. This means HPE curricula require regular renewal to ensure their content stays current. In addition, healthcare systems worldwide are chronically overburdened, in part due to an undersupply of skilled and capable clinicians and health professional educators [3, 4]. This has driven a constant search for more innovative and pedagogically sound means of delivering high-throughput and high-yield HPE curricula at scale.

As such, it is not surprising that health professional educators are increasingly embracing online education due to its potential to meet the sector's specific learning needs [5–7]. Educational technology has advanced rapidly in recent years, providing increasingly sophisticated techniques for delivering learning experiences to students [6–8]. In addition, the infrastructure to deliver these experiences has become much more widely available, notably through widespread access to high-speed broadband internet and mobile computing devices (in high-income nations, at least).

Pleasingly, alongside the increased adoption of online education techniques, educational research into the pedagogical underpinnings of these digital learning tools and techniques has also advanced to give us a far more detailed understanding of their best-practice implementation [8–10]. However, given the recency and speed of these developments, many health professional educators remain unfamiliar with the tools and techniques, their evidence base, and the practicalities of designing and delivering these learning experiences.

This introductory chapter begins by examining the definition and ways of classifying online education. It then outlines the potential opportunities for health professional educators who embrace online learning and balances this against some of the challenges of online education. It concludes with an outline of the key educational learning theories that can be applied to online learning.

1.2 Current State of Play: And How Did We Get Here?

Broadly speaking, education has always utilized multiple concurrent formats to maximize students' learning. Traditionally, this was in-person classes/lectures supplemented by textbooks (written-text). The combination of these formats was seen to synergistically aid in the learning process and has been used across all age groups and settings [11, 12].

With the advancement of technology, new devices added to the potential educational formats that could be used. Analog media devices such as the tape-deck, radio and TV enabled the production of basic audio and visual learning formats [13, 14]. These were subject to a variety of limitations including minimal personalisation, lack of feedback, production costs, and access issues. Thus, they were mainly used as supplementary learning techniques, with face-to-face teaching remaining the primary format.

Analog formats were progressively superseded by digital formats (text-on-screen, MP3s, digital video), and widespread commercial availability of personal computers (PC) began the convergence of all these formats onto a single device – with written text, audio, visual, and active-learning exercises all able to be delivered by a PC [15, 16] (**See** Table 1.1).

In addition, technological advancements in PC processing power and software development meant that, throughout the 1990s, increasingly sophisticated and pedagogically driven digital learning materials became more widely available [17, 18]. However, despite this, the lack of connection to an instructor remained a major deficit in Digital Learning. As such, Digital Learning continued to occupy the supplementary role in most educational experiences.

The advent of the internet began a major change in this situation. Internet access would provide the means to digitally bridge the gap between the instructor and student [19, 20], removing the need for physical proximity, which had been one of the most significant rate-limiting steps that kept face-to-face learning as the premier teaching modality.

However, even with this major hurdle removed, the move to online learning was neither universal nor rapid. Familiarity and experience with the more traditional face-to-face teaching models meant both learners and the educational community were relatively slow to engage in online learning for formal education [21].

Nevertheless, in 2020, the COVID-19 pandemic resulted in a rapid and, in most cases, mandatory transition to online delivery of HPE courses worldwide [6, 22]. The negligible lead time to do this meant that planned, orderly transitions into online teaching were the exception rather than the rule. Luckily, the technological infrastructure in the form of broadband internet, video-conferencing software and learning management systems already existed to facilitate this change. However, the acquisition, staff upskilling, and implementation of these were generally enacted in an ad hoc manner driven by expedience [23, 24]. The resultant learner experience of online teaching was thus inconsistent [24, 25].

Table 1.1 Timeline of major HPE advances

Year	Pedagogical advancement	Technological innovation
1960s	Simulated and standardized patients	
1970s	Objective structured clinical examination	
	Student-centred learning	
	Active learning (problem based learning)	
	Case specificity of clinical expertise	
1980s	Progress testing	Personal computing
	Key-feature items to assess clinical competence	
1990–1994	Clinical teacher knowledge and reasoning	Learning management systems
	Longitudinal integrated clerkships	Laptop computing
	The hidden curriculum	
	Competency based education	
	Experience based learning	
1995–1999	Mini clinical evaluation exercise/360 degree assessment	Internet publicly available
	Teaching and assessing professionalism	Wi-Fi launched
	Interprofessional education	
	Social accountability of health professionals	
2000–2004	Entrustable professional activities	Social media
	Programmatic assessment	Simulation technology
	Reflective practice	Broadband internet
	Inter and multidisciplinary education	
2005–2009	Correlating education to clinical outcomes	Smartphones
		4G launched
2010–2014	Microlearning	Tablet computers
		Videoconferencing
		HTML5 package (H5P)
2015–2019		Virtual reality
		Augmented reality
2020		Artificial intelligence

With the major health impacts of the COVID-19 pandemic now behind us, the emerging HPE landscape is a heterogeneous one. Learners' attitudes and expectations around online education have changed. Having experienced the flexibility of online delivery, there is now a strong expectation this will continue, and learners are often reluctant to return to lecture halls [26]. Conversely, educators are still not uniformly enthusiastic about online education, and large portions of the sector remain unfamiliar with online best practices, its evidence base, and the practicalities of designing and delivering these learning experiences [27].

1.3 Defining Online Education

Before diving into an exploration of Online Education, it is important, firstly, to agree on what is meant by this term as many potential definitions exist in the educational community [28].

We advocate a simple definition as follows:

> **Online Education** - Any form of education that is enabled or facilitated by the internet

This definition of online learning is intentionally broad to be as inclusive as possible. It thus encompasses the vast range of online learning experiences that can be designed and delivered (further discussed in Sect. 1.4).

Another, important second term is also worth defining here.

> **Digital Education** – Any form of education that is enabled by digital means

In the current educational landscape, these two terms have become effectively interchangeable as digital education is almost universally enabled or facilitated in some way by the Internet. However, it is worth noting the semantic difference between the two terms, as, in the strictest sense, digital education does not absolutely require an online element.

While both terms will be used in this book, the predominant focus will be on Online Education.

1.4 Classifying Online Education

The need for common terminology when discussing online education becomes apparent when we consider the number of potential permutations of online delivery that exist. Means et al. identified nine pedagogical dimensions by which online educational programs can be classified in their design [29], a typology which was further refined by Hodges et al. [30] (Table 1.2).

Beyond these pedagogical features, there are also further program factors that must be considered. These are its context, size, resourcing, and the specific learning tools that will be utilised to achieve its pedagogical aims.

Best-practice online educational design means considering the pedagogical domains as well as the further program factors to design a fit-for-purpose learning experience for your target group of learners.

Table 1.2 Online learning pedagogical domains – adapted from Means et al. [29] and Hodges et al. [30]

Pedagogical domain	Classifications
Instructor role	Online Active instruction online Small presence online None
Student role	Online Listen/read/view Complete problems or answer questions Explore simulation and resources Collaborate with peers
Core pedagogy	Expository Practice Exploratory Collaborative
Student-instructor ratio	<35 to 1 36–99 to 1 100–999 to 1 >1000 to 1
Modality	Fully online Blended (over 50% online) Blended (25–50% online) Web-enabled face-to-face (F2F)
Online communication synchrony	Asynchronous only Synchronous only Some blend of both
Pacing	Self-paced (open entry, open exit) Class-paced Class-paced with some self-paced
Role of online assessments	Determine if student is ready for new content Tell system how to support the student (adaptive instruction) Provide student or teacher with information about learning state Input to grade Identify students at risk of failure
Source of feedback	Automated Teacher Peers

1.5 Opportunities

Online education has numerous qualitative points of difference that are either not possible in face-to-face models or are expedited through digital delivery. By leveraging these inherent strengths there is the opportunity to significantly augment already existing training programs and, in some cases, create a whole new class of learning experiences.

1.5.1 Enhanced Flexibility, Accessibility and Convenience

Flexible learning refers to educational methods that allow a user to learn when they want, how they want, and what they want [31]. This is clearly a desirable characteristic for health professionals who are typically time-poor [32] and may have intermittent and unpredictable windows of opportunity for educational activities.

Online education is an effective means for overcoming the barrier of timing. Asynchronous teaching tasks allow learners to control their learning environment for optimal results [33, 34] and provide flexibility in managing their learning schedules [35, 36].

Additionally, online education removes the need for physical proximity. It provides multiple potential communication channels for diverse and effective interaction between instructor and learner [37, 38], hence removing a major rate-limiting step and allowing educational relationships to be formed between individuals in any corner of the globe. Simultaneously, it removes costs involved with in-person travel to training, such as costs of flights, petrol, childcare and time away from work [39, 40].

In doing so, it vastly improves the accessibility of learning materials to the benefit of all learners, but especially for those who live remotely or internationally.

1.5.2 Breadth (Through Accessibility)

A byproduct of increasing accessibility is increasing the viability of previously 'niche' programs. This is particularly relevant in HPE, given areas of subspecialty may only have very small numbers of practitioners. Therefore, attracting enough learners to a face-to-face program in a specific physical location is difficult, often making the economics and overall benefit of devising and delivering an educational program questionable.

Online programming means the educational cohort can be situated anywhere in the world. This allows for the aggregation of otherwise disparate learners, making more programs feasible from both an educational and economic perspective, ultimately increasing the diversity of potential educational topics and programs [41].

1.5.3 Scalability

Scalability refers to the ability of an educational program to expand and cater to increased demand. Traditional face-to-face educational programs are typically restricted in scalability for a variety of reasons – for instance, limitations in staffing (i.e., a limited amount of qualified teaching faculty), in physical space (i.e., a classroom/lecture theatre can only accommodate up to a certain size), in timing, (i.e., everyone must be present at the same time) and issues with diminished educational experiences with larger class sizes.

Online education has the potential to overcome all these issues because it is not constrained to a physical (or temporal) location, and many learning experiences do not require live (synchronous) interaction with faculty staff. In addition, there can be automation of assessment. As a result, online programs are highly scalable, as best demonstrated in Massive Open Online Courses (MOOCs), and large-scale, open-access online learning programs [42, 43].

1.5.4 Environmental Sustainability

Online education reduces the need for consumables, catering, and travel and can, therefore, minimise the impact on the environment through the reduction of landfill and carbon emissions. Dudian et al. [41] measured the impact of printed materials alone and showed the transition to online learning made a measurable impact on the CO_2 footprint of each learner, thus improving the overall environmental sustainability of the learning process.

1.5.5 Personalised Learning

Online education allows for personalised learning experiences catering to individual students' needs and interests [44]. Adaptive learning technologies can track learner progress and provide personalised feedback and recommendations – often instantaneously. There is also the ability for smart learning programs to be able to modify learning activities in real-time to adjust to the performance and inputs of the learner [45, 46]. In addition, the nature of the platform gives learners the flexibility to spend time reflecting, processing, and researching further where they deem it appropriate [47].

These kinds of adaptive learning activities are inherently tailored to the individual and provide a higher level of personalisation than most in-person experiences, where an instructor's attention must be divided between many learners. This is particularly beneficial in HPE, where learners of multidisciplinary backgrounds and varying levels of pre-existing knowledge may undertake a learning program, making 'one-size-fits-all' approaches unfit for purpose.

1.5.6 Collaborative and Multidisciplinary Learning Experiences

It is increasingly clear that, to be effective, HPE must reflect the realities of everyday clinical practice, where health practitioners work cooperatively in a multidisciplinary environment. This maximises clinical effectiveness by combining complementary areas of expertise and thus being able to deliver wholistic healthcare to each patient. Therefore, individually 'siloed' learning opportunities, where different health disciplines train independently of one another, are rapidly becoming outdated.

Online education provides a great opportunity for the integration of HPE learning in a multidisciplinary (and interprofessional) setting. The flexibility of learning management systems and the modular composition of different learning activities lend themselves well to transverse integration of learning across disciplines. Students and faculty can interact via a variety of means, including discussion boards, live chats, and virtual classrooms. These tools foster an environment of active learning and have been demonstrated to be an effective platform for forming relationships, which enriches the learning experience and can be sustained even beyond the completion of the program [48].

Online education can also facilitate learners to view issues from multiple angles (both literally and metaphorically) and thus facilitate more insightful, well-rounded opinions on educational topics [49, 50].

1.5.7 Data-Driven Decision Making

Digital learning significantly streamlines the collection of data at both a macro and micro level. These can then be used to measure student performance, identify areas of improvement, and make data-driven decisions to optimise future learning experiences for individual learners.

Moreover, analytics can inform strategic decisions at an institutional level, guiding the development of courses, allocation of resources, and overall educational strategies. This ensures that enhancements are based on data [51] and not dependent on potentially flawed or incomplete evaluations.

1.5.8 Advanced Visualisation and Simulation

Recent advances in educational technology have allowed forms of highly sophisticated visualisation, allowing concepts and structures to be depicted in ways that were previously impossible. For instance, representation of complex cell processes is possible in animated environments that would otherwise have been explained verbally or through static images [7, 52].

In addition, while visualisations can be used for imparting knowledge – a key component of HPE curricula is training health professionals to perform a wide range of practical and procedural tasks. Advanced simulation techniques, including the use of virtual reality, are a means of being able to create an environment to learn such psychomotor skills [50]. This goes hand in hand with gamified learning techniques and emerging technologies such as augmented reality. As these technologies mature and the cost to develop and deliver training via these platforms decreases, their applications in HPE are only likely to grow.

1.6 Challenges of Online Education

Online education does come with challenges that must be carefully considered and accounted for when implementing a new online HPE program. Technological limitations, such as internet bandwidth issues, software and hardware constraints, and potential privacy and security concerns are particularly noteworthy [53, 54]. Costs, development time, maintenance and renewal, the need for specialised development teams, and the need for continual faculty development and training further compound these challenges from an educational organisation perspective.

Learners face issues such as limitations in self-efficacy [55], environmental distractions, lack of dedicated study areas, multitasking difficulties, language proficiency, technical proficiency, reduced enjoyment, and motivation, often struggling to engage deeply with the material. It is also possible that online learning can leave learners feeling disconnected and fatigued, contributing to a reduced sense of community and identity, isolation, and disengagement [56, 57]. Furthermore, it may not be as conducive to dealing with sensitive or confronting material, with some documented examples of learners feeling reticent to be vulnerable in the online setting and educators finding it difficult to overcome this [58].

Internationally, there are regional differences in baseline technological proficiency and technology availability that make some areas less susceptible to adopt online education [59]. Depending on the structure of the online activity, the lack of direct face-to-face social interaction and knowledge exchange may contribute to higher attrition rates, leaving students feeling isolated and less supported. This may have contributed to findings in some studies that graduation rates from online programs are often lower than those of in-person courses [60, 61].

Learners and educators have also shown some reticence in embracing online educational techniques. For educators, it has been shown that their attitudes towards online education are heavily influenced by institutional culture, the educator's own knowledge, skills, and belief in the medium, their commitment to professional development, and their connection with the learners [53]. Learners also show varying levels of enthusiasm [62], and these are governed by factors that include their own technology savviness, their perception of its usefulness, and their need for convenience [63].

Despite these challenges, improvements in student support systems and thoughtfully constructed, learner-centred course designs are potential solutions that can overcome many of these issues to enhance the effectiveness and appeal of online education.

1.7 When Is the Right Time to Go Online?

It is always too early for rigorous evaluation (of a new technique) until, unfortunately, it is suddenly too late – Health Economist Martin Buxton, 1987 [64]

While there are some educators who advocate such a change should only occur when the evidence conclusively demonstrates that the new technique improves educational outcomes, this does not represent real-life practice, and likely not even best practice.

The most widespread approach to curricula renewal is 'evidence-informed' decision-making [65] (note the contrast to 'evidence-based' decision-making). This is characterised by the *preference* to enact educational interventions that have documented evidence of their effect, but, where this does not exist, the acceptance that an intervention can still be rationally implemented where there is a demonstrable educational gap, and there is an intervention with a sound theoretical basis that can fill that gap [65–68].

When one looks at such headline pedagogies as Problem-Based Learning [69] and Competency-Based Education [70], these are examples of times when the integration of a new teaching technique into curricula preceded the generation of evidence around them [71, 72]. In both cases, there was a clear deficiency noted in current training systems at the time of inception, and the new pedagogy was applied to rectify them.

While this may be surprising at first – particularly to health professional practitioners who, in their clinical work, have been systemically taught to adhere to the principles of evidence-based practice (EBP) – it is erroneous to apply the same rules of EBP from clinical care directly into HPE. Although there are many similarities, there are also some key divergences. Educational science has no equivalent 'preclinical' stage where you can test a theory in a lab. The first phase of an educational trial, following a sound theoretical basis, must be a trial in an actual teaching environment.

Therefore, although there remain vocal proponents for restraint in the application of new teaching techniques [66, 70], this is a relatively conservative approach and actually leaves educators and educational institutions at risk of succumbing to Buxton's law, which is to paraphrase, "it's always too early to implement until it's suddenly too late".

When it comes to online education, the inflection point between 'too early' and 'too late' has arguably already passed. COVID-19 unequivocally demonstrated the utility of an online approach and, perhaps more importantly, its feasibility. Changing educational 'norms' and 'set beliefs' is perhaps one of the most difficult aspects of any change implementation. However, the mandatory nature of virtual education during the COVID years has given the impetus for educational change that may have otherwise arrived much more gradually. This has also created a more fertile landscape for change due to increased resourcing for technological infrastructure, upskilling in technical literacy (through mandatory usage), and redefining learners' expectations in terms of what level of flexibility and accessibility could be reasonably expected when undertaking HPE.

Thus, it is incumbent upon health professional educators to proactively be incorporating online education into their formal curricula and building authentically designed learning experiences that leverage the benefits of the medium to their utmost while similarly accounting for its potential deficiencies. To do this requires a familiarity with the principles of sound curricular design.

1.8 Meaningful Design in Online Education

To meaningfully design online education, it is important to first consider some key truisms (i.e., indisputable facts) that must be considered in any online HPE design.

(a) *There are many online delivery contexts. Each of these inherently varies from traditional face-to-face teaching and has individually exploitable strengths and weaknesses.*

Online education is not a homogenous experience. Means' pedagogical classification demonstrates that there are dozens of different structural permutations of how online learning may be delivered. Beyond these structural differences, there are also significant *contextual differences* in which education is delivered. For instance, social media, Massive Open Online Courses (MOOCs), short courses, symposia, conferences, and even tertiary award courses such as degrees and certifications.

The learners in each of these delivery contexts will be quite different, and one must design the delivered learning experience to cater for these differences. An overall approach to curriculum design, including worked examples, is described in Chap. 2 - **Designing effective, online health professional curricula**.

In addition, educators must also understand how to consider and account for the different online educational contexts. This will be explored in further detail in Chap. 3 – **Contexts and conditions for online learning success**.

(b) *Effective online education is delivered in qualitatively different ways from face-to-face learning.*

During the rapid move of HPE programs online during COVID-19, many students felt that learning experiences were not commensurate with face-to-face delivery [24]. Yet, this was not necessarily a balanced comparison. The rapid online transition generally meant often that only the most simplistic form of learning design was enacted – where the pre-existing in-person activity was directly transposed onto a screen, either via video-conferencing software or lecture capture [73, 74]. This form of learning design leverages none of the natural strengths of online learning nor takes into account its natural weaknesses. As was best expressed by Hodges: "Well-planned online learning experiences are meaningfully different from courses offered online in response to a crisis or disaster." [30].

Delivery methods that are fit-for-purpose in the online environment are discussed in detail in Chap. 4 – **Best practice design and delivery of digital learning tools and techniques** and online teaching and facilitation methods in Chap. 5 - **Teaching and facilitating online learning**.

In addition to these truisms, online HPE provides a perfect opportunity to design forward-looking curricula that will embrace emerging trends in the healthcare and educational fields. One of these is the previously mentioned opportunity of providing multidisciplinary learning experiences that are reflective of real-world healthcare scenarios. A detailed exploration of how this can be integrated into online curricula is covered in Chap. 6 - **Multidisciplinary and interprofessional education in the online environment.** This is followed by a discussion of another important emerging influence, artificial intelligence (AI). Chapter 7 – **Applications of artificial intelligence to health professional education** will ensure health professional educators are primed and prepared to utilize the extraordinary capabilities of AI in their HPE curricula while also accounting for potential weaknesses it has exposed in traditional teaching methods and assessments.

Finally, actively implementing an online curriculum involves translating these learnings and applying them to each educator's individualised learning context. Chapter 8 – **Implementing and Leading Online Education Transformation** provides guidance on how to do this. Thus, this manual covers the end-to-end process of meaningful online educational design from theory to design, development and implementation.

Example of meaningful design choices in HPE

Consider a potential online short course updating on recent drug developments in melanoma, aimed at multidisciplinary health professionals with a total time commitment of 2 h, to be completed in their own time. The aim of this program is for clinicians to be able to explain to a patient the drugs' mode of action, benefits, and potential side effects.

One can first identify some of the specific learning needs of this program (highlighted in **bold**)

As the learners are busy and expected to complete this in their own time, a **flexible delivery format** would increase the likelihood of undertaking the program.

The learning outcomes for this program are for the learner to have acquired knowledge (about the drug mode of action, benefits, and side effects) and be able to perform a specific task (explain the drugs to a patient). Therefore, the educational delivery format would ideally **facilitate both knowledge and behaviour transfer.**

Given that the learners' backgrounds are multidisciplinary, the program will need to **account for large potential variance in background knowledge** of drugs, from minimal knowledge to fairly high levels of knowledge.

In addition, as the program will be delivered over a short time frame, this will need to be a **high-yield learning experience** to impart the knowledge quickly and effectively.

Then, one should meaningfully design a program that accounts for each of these needs. A potential format may be:

- Online, asynchronous learning platform – to account for the need for flexible delivery.
- Information is delivered in short videos and infographics – to facilitate knowledge transfer and be a high-yield learning experience.
- Incorporation of self-testing to encourage both knowledge and behaviour transfer.
- Modular, self-paced design to account for differences in initial knowledge level.

1.9 Core Educational Theories that Can Be Applied to Online Education

All learning is ultimately a cognitive exercise that is regulated by the innate ways in which the human brain processes information. 'Optimizing learning' is, in effect, trying to create learning experiences that align with how the human brain processes and retains information to ensure it can do this in the most efficient and effective way possible.

For centuries, educators and educational psychologists have been trying to understand these innate processing methods of the brain. Many theories have been proposed to explain these. These are called learning theories.

A good understanding of learning theories allows us to effectively leverage the strengths of online education by designing learning experiences that align with the ways that our brain thinks. Here we will describe several key learning theories that can be utilized by educators to enhance knowledge acquisition and application in the online arena. These are discussed below and a summary of these is listed in Table 1.3.

1.9.1 Cognitive Load Theory

Cognitive Load Theory (CLT) explains how information is perceived and processed through different memory "compartments". Each of these memory compartments serves a different purpose and has different capacities [75].

Table 1.3 Summary of learning theories relevant to online education and their design implications

Educational theory	Key points	Implications for online educational design
Cognitive load theory	• There are three types of memory: sensory, working, long-term • There are fixed-rate pathways between these memory compartments • These fixed-rate pathways can be overwhelmed	• Ensure information is adequately paced to avoid overwhelming memory capacity • Self-paced learning activities (e.g. through asynchronous activities and modularization) reduce risk of overwhelming memory processing conduits
'Dual coding' theory (multimedia learning theory)	• The human brain processes information by two channels: auditory and visual • These have separate fixed-rate processing capacities	• Providing multimedia learning experiences (utilising both channels e.g. video) maximizes learning efficiency
Constructivism theory	• Learners construct new knowledge by progressively connecting new information with what already exists in their mental frameworks	• Aim to design iterative educational experiences that progressively build and extend upon previous material • Learning methods that encourage exploration, critical thinking and active knowledge construction (e.g. collaborative projects, interactive simulations) are well suited to this
Social learning theory	• All learning occurs in a social context through observation, role modelling, imitation and social interactions	• Fostering social interactions between learners as well as between learners and instructors should be facilitated wherever possible (e.g. through use of discussion forums, group activities, synchronous video meetings, webinars etc)
Connectivism theory	• 'Learning' occurs through the formation of connections between 'nodes' which may be people, technological, physical or metaphysical constructs • Its emphasis is on the process of connection formation	• Education can provide a means of connecting the large and diverse amounts of information and experiences found online into meaningful knowledge • Online technologies such as social media, wikis, discussion boards, zoom etc. can be leveraged to connect these 'nodes'

(continued)

Table 1.3 (continued)

Educational theory	Key points	Implications for online educational design
Experiential learning theory	• Learning is continuous and dynamic • It is obtained through experiences	• This is exploitable through active online learning techniques such as simulation, virtual reality and gamification
Adult learning theory (andragogy)	• Adults learn in different ways to children • They are independent, self-directed, problem-oriented, practical and are self-motivated	• Incorporate opportunities for self-paced learning and learner choice • Ensure clear connection between learning and its practical application
Actor-network theory (ANT)	• ANT is closely related to connectivism in that it looks at the relationship and connections between people and things • ANT is not a learning theory per se, but rather a social theory • Its emphasis is on understanding the networks (as a whole) rather than on the connections	• Online educational design should consider all learners in the 'network' and in maintaining and building these collective networks • This can be achieved through collaborative learning experiences such as discussion forums, group activities, synchronous video meetings, webinars etc
Transformative learning theory	• In the process of learning, pivotal events or realisations can fundamentally alter leaners' self-perceptions, worldviews and future actions	• Online education has the ability to bring about transformative realisation that can make lifelong impacts on learners thereafter • Educators should be empowered to address critically important topics for health professionals such as inclusivity, discernment, openness, resilience, and reflection

- There is the initial 'sensory' memory, which is momentary and fleeting. It is the immediate experience of the stimulus and is rapidly displaced by further stimuli.
- A portion of the sensory memory passes through to be stored into the 'working memory.' This has a limited capacity (generally 7 items ±2), and items can be stored for roughly a minute or less (e.g., a phone number which can be retained for a short period until it is written down but unlikely to be recalled the next day).
- Finally, there is the long-term memory. This has a virtually unlimited capacity, and knowledge held within it is potentially permanent. The ultimate goal of all education is for information to be successfully stored herein.

Memories must be transferred from the working into the long-term memory through a specific encoding and storage process, which we would colloquially term 'learning' (Fig. 1.1) Different pedagogical techniques drive this process, such as 'active learning', 'reflection and 'associative learning.'

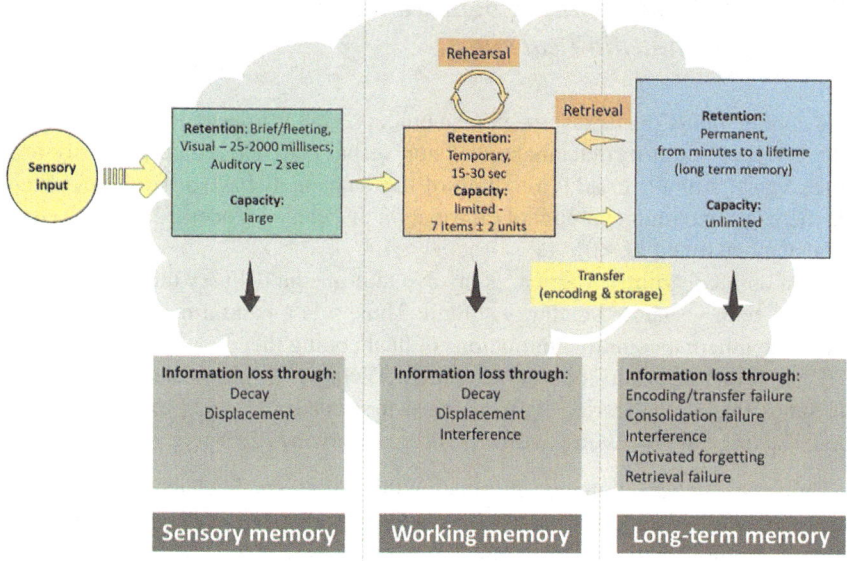

Fig. 1.1 Three-stage model of human memory - From Kok et al. [76]

Cognitive load theory (CLT) suggests there are several fixed, rate-limiting steps along the way to long-term storage, which may lead to inefficiency – or breakdown – of the learning process if not properly accounted for. The most notable of these is the capacity of the working memory. This is relatively limited and can very easily be inadvertently overloaded. If we remain with the telephone number analogy, after the first 7 digits, working memory can be overwhelmed within seconds. A 15-digit number will almost never be retained and, in fact, may cause greater confusion as one attempts to cram this information into working memory, causing information loss on both ends. In most cases, learners would be better off attempting to only remember the first 7 digits and make no attempt at remembering the other 8, because when a learner attempts to remember all 15 digits it increases the likelihood of misremembering all 15 [77, 78].

Therefore, good learning a) design allows for information to be presented in chunks that are small enough to be reliably held within the working memory for the length of time it takes for this information to be successfully encoded and stored into the long-term memory, and b) paces all activities to not be at a speed that is greater than the likely 'forward egress' of information into long-term memory.

Finally, this speed of egress is directly correlated with the quality of the pedagogical learning design. More effective learning techniques allow more rapid information movement into the long-term memory, as do techniques such as regular revisitation of material to enhance consolidation, use of appropriate intermissions to reset working memory and retrieval practice to accustomise the brain to being able to relocate the information when required.

1.9.2 The 'Dual Coding' Cognitive Theory of Multimedia Learning

Dual coding theory posits that the human brain processes information via two channels: a verbal (auditory) channel and a non-verbal channel, which primarily processes visual stimuli. In addition, both of these channels have a fixed bandwidth, i.e., there is a maximum amount of information that can be processed via each channel at any one time [79, 80].

Most online learning experiences involve multimedia delivery through a combination of both visual and auditory stimuli. Thus, it is a natural medium that overcomes the inherent cognitive limitations of dual coding theory.

Thus, following from this, the Cognitive Theory of Multimedia Learning [17, 81] states that by delivering well-designed multimedia learning experiences that capitalise on both processing pathways, one can provide a learning experience that:

1. Delivers a higher volume of information than either single channel could alone
2. Produces synergistic learning (whereby information provided on each channel provides information that explicates what is being conveyed via the alternate route)

As such, online education that delivers information in multimedia formats is highly preferable to any single delivery method (e.g., plain text on screen or audio only) and leverages multimedia learning theory to its maximum effect for the benefit of the learner (Fig. 1.2).

1.9.3 Constructivism Theory

In constructivism, learners construct knowledge by connecting new information that they learn with what already exists in their own mental frameworks. Context is perceived through the interaction with the learner and not as an extrinsic or intrinsic environment. It is also unpredictably and constantly changing depending on the perception of the learner and interactions with the learning materials and other stakeholders involved. This theoretical approach encourages exploration, engagement, critical thinking, problem-solving and active knowledge construction through the integration of online discussion forums, collaborative projects, and interactive simulations integrated into online learning platforms [83].

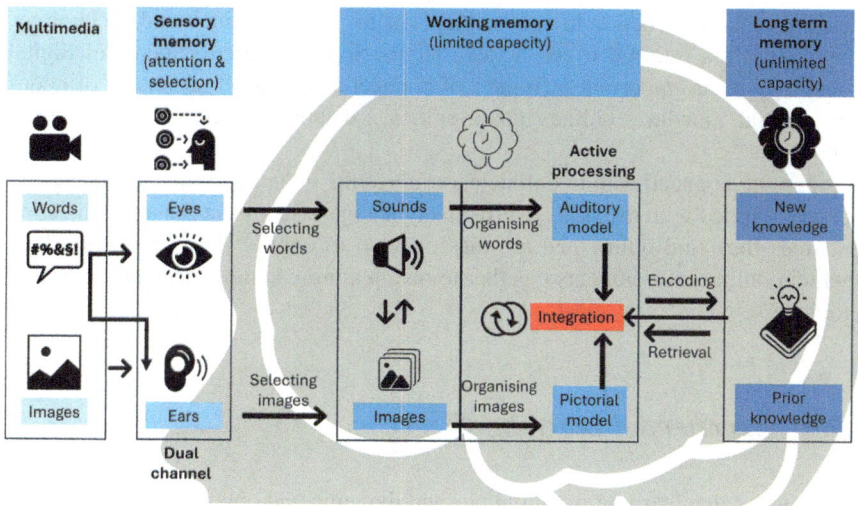

Fig. 1.2 Multimedia Learning Theory. Multimedia learning is an active process consisting of a combination of words and images that are interpreted via sensory memory. It is processed by two channels (auditory and visual), which have finite capacity but can be used simultaneously. The working memory organises these sounds and images and integrates them together with prior knowledge from long-term memory; this is then encoded into long-term memory (adapted from Krumm et al. [82])

1.9.4 Social Learning Theory

Social learning theory was initially described by Albert Bandura who posited that humans primarily learn through observation, role modelling, imitation and social interactions. In other words, all learning occurs in a social context, and therefore, socialisation is pivotal for an individual to learn. The social context is an important part of online education contexts, even if, or especially if, learners are physically separated. This theory highlights the importance of generating ideas, perspectives, and feedback by fostering social interactions, discussion forums, and group activities within the learner cohort [84].

1.9.5 Connectivism Theory

Connectivism is an innovative learning theory that stipulates that learners should embrace the integration of thoughts, theories, and information. It promotes the role of group dynamics, networks, connections, collaborations, and open dialogue to enhance decision-making, problem-solving and understanding complex concepts. Connectivism shares some common ground with social learning theory, but the connections it describes need not only to be between people but can also include metaphysical constructs and non-sentient items like machines and technology. These are often referred to as 'nodes'. Connectivism explicitly identifies digital technology as an important facilitator of connections through its variety of nodes e.g., social media, online communities, databases and communication technologies.

Applying connectivism to online learning results in an approach where learners can be equipped with the skills to effectively navigate and make sense of education resources they find online and are thus enabled to connect the information they obtain in online environments together to obtain a more complete understanding of a topic [85].

1.9.6 Experiential Learning Theory

Kolb posited that learning is continuous and dynamic and obtained through experiences. He described this as understanding being 'created through the transformation of experience' [86]. He describes two ways of grasping experience in Experiential Learning Theory, through abstract conceptualisation and concrete experience. Online learning contexts can provide opportunities for learners to apply theoretical knowledge in practical scenarios through the integration of simulations, case studies, virtual labs, and real-world projects.

1.9.7 Adult Learning Theory (Andragogy)

Adult Learning Theory was proposed by Knowles, who suggested that adults learn in different ways to children. It has several core assumptions:

- Self-concept: Adults have a self-concept that is independent and self-directed.
- Experience: Adults accumulate a reservoir of experiences that serve as a resource for learning.
- Readiness to learn: Adults become ready to learn when they perceive a need to know or solve a problem.
- Orientation to learning: Adults are oriented to learning that is practical and problem-centered rather than subject-centered.
- Motivation: Adults are motivated to learn by internal factors, such as intrinsic interests and self-esteem, rather than external rewards [87].

Some aspects of this learning theory are disputed, with commentators suggesting that what Knowles was describing was an ideal state for adult learners rather than a set of universal truisms [88]. However, it is fair to say that many adults do share these learning characteristics, and therefore they should be considered in HPE education which is focussed on adults. Incorporating opportunities for self-paced learning, learner choice, and the ability to connect new knowledge with real-life experiences can thus be useful techniques on online HPE.

1.9.8 Actor-Network Theory (ANT)

ANT views online learning contexts as intricate networks of interconnected actors, including learners, educators, digital tools and technologies, and institutions. This theoretical perspective believes that all these elements have agency and influence the dynamics of learning. To promote equitable and inclusive online education, digital divide issues must be addressed, providing support for all actors in the network, and adapting the learning materials to suit the online environment [89].

1.9.9 Transformative Learning Theory

Transformative learning, as originally outlined by Mezirow [90], describes how pivotal events or realisations can fundamentally alter our self-perception, worldview, and subsequent actions. As such, the process of learning is effectively revealing new ways of thinking, thus 'transforming' their perspective. Incorporating a transformative learning lens to online education is a powerful method to impact the views and actions of learners. In addition, it can assist in promoting inclusivity, discernment, openness, resilience, and reflection – all of which are vital skills in HPE. A more detailed exploration of transformative learning and its application to online education is covered in Chap. 5 – **Teaching and Facilitating Online.**

1.10 'Online Education' or Just 'Education'?

Although this book is explicitly about the techniques and best-practice application of Online Education, this is not meant to imply that Online Education is a distinct, mutually exclusive entity that sits as an alternative to Traditional Education.

In any given era, the primary, inherent responsibility of an educator is to facilitate learners to learn. Naturally, they will utilise the tools/devices/technology that exist to try and ensure the most efficient and effective learning experience possible. Many major new devices have been introduced over the centuries that have presented educators with new opportunities to improve the learning experience. The pen, book, typewriter, televisions, calculators, PowerPoint, the tape recorder… all of these provided new, qualitatively different methods of delivering education. When initially introduced, all of these seemed era-defining at the time, but in retrospect, now they appear to be a natural and inherent part of educational delivery that are there to be used when the learning context requires it.

Similarly, online education is a tool that - while new and novel at this moment – does not necessarily represent a complete invalidation of all educational processes that have come before. Rather, they represent a new suite of tools that will be widely used **in addition** to other tested and time-proven teaching techniques. Some programs may have minimal benefit from the implementation of online education techniques, but many others will have vast potential benefits.

This manual should be of equal use no matter what end of the spectrum your current teaching curriculum falls into. However, it should not be mistaken to imply that all educational curricula must, or should, utilise all of the principles described. Instead, it should prompt a judicious individualised consideration of whether the pedagogical and/or logistical benefits of an online education technique are worth incorporating into (or supplanting) existing curriculum components.

1.11 Tips and Tricks

- It is normal that different educators will embrace online education with varying levels of enthusiasm and at different rates. Implementation approaches that make the effort to cultivate true 'buy-in' by educational colleagues will ultimately lead to better working environments (and outcomes) than rigid, hard-line approaches.
- Although there are many opportunities afforded by online education, be strategic and deliberate in choosing the ones that are suitable and desirable for your specific context. It may make more sense to lean into one or two rather than trying to generate a program that leverages all of them but only superficially.
- Online education is sometimes seen incorrectly as a way of being able to deliver education cheaply. This is not universally true and is a pitfall that should be avoided. Like all education, good online learning programs come at a cost, and the quality of a program will depend on the investment placed into it.
- The 'online' vs 'traditional education' dichotomy tends to be more arbitrarily divisive than it is helpful. Encourage colleagues to see moving online as part of a natural, ongoing evolution of education rather than an abrupt reconfiguration of the learning world.

1.12 Conclusion

Online Education is a format that is well suited to HPE due to a combination of features, including flexibility, accessibility, yield, and personalisation ability. As such, programs have much to gain by capitalizing on these opportunities and embracing online delivery, either in part or in full. To do this effectively means taking a considered approach to online curriculum design, which, in turn, relies upon leveraging several core educational theories that lend themselves towards online learning. Educators who do this will position themselves well in the rapidly evolving landscape of HPE.

References

1. Fontelo P, Liu F. A review of recent publication trends from top publishing countries. Syst Rev. 2018;7(1):147.
2. Akiki V, Troussard X, Metges JP, Devos P. Global trends in oncology research: a mixed-methods study of publications and clinical trials from 2010 to 2019. Cancer Rep. 2023;6(1):e1650.
3. Ahmed H, Ahmed H, Ahmed H, Ahmed H, Carmody J, Carmody JB. On the looming physician shortage and strategic expansion of graduate medical education. Cureus. 2020;12(7)
4. American Association of Medical Colleges. The complexities of physician supply and demand: projections from 2021 to 2036 [Internet]. 2024 [cited 2024 May 25]. Available from: https://www.aamc.org/media/75236/download?attachment
5. Wozniak H, Ellaway R, de Jong PGM. What have we learnt about using digital technologies in health professional education. Med J Aust. 2018;209(10):431–3.
6. Jeffries PR, Bushardt RL, DuBose-Morris R, Hood C, Kardong-Edgren S, Pintz C, et al. The role of technology in health professions education during the COVID-19 pandemic. Acad Med. 2021;
7. Kok DL, Dushyanthen S, Peters GW, Sapkaroski D, Barrett M, Sim J, et al. Screen-based digital learning methods in radiation oncology and medical education. Tech Innov Patient Support Radiat Oncol. 2022;24:86–93.
8. Masters K, Correia R, Nemethy K, Benjamin J, Carver TE, MacNeill H. Online learning in health professions education. Part 2: tools and practical application: AMEE guide No. 163. Med Teach. 2023:1–16.
9. Chen BY, Kern DE, Kearns RM, Thomas PA, Hughes MT, Tackett S. From modules to MOOCs: application of the six-step approach to online curriculum development for medical education. Acad Med. 2019;94(5):678–85.
10. Roach VA, Attardi SM. Twelve tips for applying Moore's theory of transactional distance to optimize online teaching. Med Teach. 2022;44(8):859–65.
11. Johansson M. Teaching mathematics with textbooks: a classroom and curricular perspective. Luleå tekniska universitet; 2006.
12. Sun Y, Kulm G, Capraro MM. Middle grade teachers' use of textbooks and their classroom instruction. J Math Educ. 2009;2(2):20–37.
13. Pavlov R, Paneva D. Interactive TV-based learning, models and standards. In: HUBUSKA Open Workshop Semantic Web and Knowledge Technologies, (pp 70–99) Varna. 2006. p. 40
14. Benschoter RP, Charles DC. Retention of classroom and television learning. J Appl Psychol. 1957;41(4):253.
15. Berk RA. Multimedia teaching with video clips: TV, movies, YouTube, and mtvU in the college classroom. Int J Technol Teach Learn. 2009;5(1)
16. Maag M. Podcasting and MP3 players: emerging education technologies. CIN Comput Inform Nurs. 2006;24(1):9–13.
17. Mayer RE, Mayer RE. The Cambridge handbook of multimedia learning: principles for reducing extraneous processing in multimedia learning : coherence, signaling, redundancy, spatial contiguity, and temporal contiguity principles; 2005. p. 183–200.
18. Moos D. Examining hypermedia learning: the role of cognitive load and self-regulated learning. J Educ Multimed Hypermedia. 2013;22(1):39–61.
19. Zhang H, Lin L, Zhan Y, Ren Y. The impact of teaching presence on online engagement behaviors. J Educ Comput Res. 2016;54(7):887–900.

20. Instructor presence in video lectures: The role of dynamic drawings, eye contact, and instructor visibility. Vol. 111. US: American Psychological Association; 2019
21. Dufner S. Reluctance toward online teaching. 2018;
22. Arday J. Covid-19 and higher education: the times they are A'Changin. Educ Rev. 2022;74(3):365–77.
23. García-Morales VJ, Garrido-Moreno A, Martín-Rojas R. The transformation of higher education after the COVID disruption: emerging challenges in an online learning scenario. Front Psychol. 2021;12:616059.
24. Rudolph J, Tan S, Crawford J, Butler-Henderson K. Perceived quality of online learning during COVID-19 in higher education in Singapore: perspectives from students, lecturers, and academic leaders. Educ Res Policy Pract. 2022;
25. Taher TMJ, Saadi RB, Oraibi RR, Ghazi HF, Abdul-Rasool S, Tuma F. E-learning satisfaction and barriers in unprepared and resource-limited systems during the COVID-19 pandemic. Cureus. 2022;14(5):e24969.
26. Emahiser J, Nguyen J, Vanier C, Sadik A. Study of live lecture attendance, student perceptions and expectations. Med Sci Educ. 2021;31(2):697–707.
27. Daniel M, Gordon M, Patricio M, Hider A, Pawlik C, Bhagdev R, et al. An update on developments in medical education in response to the COVID-19 pandemic: a BEME scoping review: BEME Guide No. 64. Med Teach. 2021;43(3):253–71.
28. Singh V, Singh V, Thurman AC. How many ways can we define online learning? A systematic literature review of definitions of online learning (1988-2018). Am J Distance Educ. 2019;33(4):289–306.
29. Means B, Bakia M, Murphy R. Learning online: what research tells us about whether. When and How. 2014
30. Hodges CB, Moore S, Lockee BB, Trust T, Bond MA, Bond MA, et al. The difference between emergency remote teaching and online learning. Educ Rev. 2020;
31. Van den Brande L. Flexible and distance learning. Wiley; 1993.
32. Grunfeld E, Zitzelsberger L, Coristine M, Whelan TJ, Aspelund F, Evans WK. Job stress and job satisfaction of cancer care workers. Psychooncology. 2005;14(1):61–9.
33. Kentnor HE. Distance education and the evolution of online learning in the United States. Curric Teach Dialogue. 2015;17(1):21–34.
34. Vonderwell S, Liang X, Alderman K. Asynchronous discussions and assessment in online learning. J Res Technol Educ. 2007;39(3):309–28.
35. Poon J. Blended learning: an institutional approach for enhancing students' learning experiences. J Online Learn Teach. 2013;9(2):271.
36. Owston R, York D, Murtha S. Student perceptions and achievement in a university blended learning strategic initiative. Internet High Educ. 2013;18:38–46.
37. Miller A, Topper A, Richardson S. Suggestions for improving IPEDS distance education data collection [Internet]. US Department of Education; 2017 [cited 2023 Sep 7]. Available from: http://nces.ed.gov/pubsearch/
38. Sharma SK, Joshi A, Sharma H. A multi-analytical approach to predict the Facebook usage in higher education. Comput Hum Behav. 2016;55:340–53.
39. Christensen CM, Johnson CW, Horn MB. Disrupting class: how disruptive innovation will change the way the world learns. McGraw-Hill; 2008.
40. Maloney S, Nicklen P, Rivers G, Foo J, Ooi YY, Reeves S, et al. A cost-effectiveness analysis of blended versus face-to-face delivery of evidence-based medicine to medical students. J Med Internet Res. 2015;17(7):e4346.
41. Dudian M, Todoran TA, Popa RA. Organisational culture shifting into online learning. Virtual Learning Practices Stud Bus Econ. 2022;17(3):57–69.
42. Roberts A, LoCasale-Crouch J, Hamre B, Buckrop J. Adapting for scalability: automating the video assessment of instructional learning. Online Learn. 2017:21.
43. Julia K, Marco K. Educational scalability in MOOCs: analysing instructional designs to find best practices. Comput Educ. 2021;161:104054.

44. Hu X, Yelland N. An investigation of preservice early childhood teachers' adoption of ICT in a teaching practicum context in Hong Kong. J Early Child Teach Educ. 2017;38(3):259–74.
45. Warner DO, Nolan M, Garcia-Marcinkiewicz A, Schultz C, Warner MA, Schroeder DR, et al. Adaptive instruction and learner interactivity in online learning: a randomized trial. Adv Health Sci Educ. 2020;25:95–109.
46. Hongsuchon T, Emary IME, Hariguna T, Qhal EMA. Assessing the impact of online-learning effectiveness and benefits in knowledge management, the antecedent of online-learning strategies and motivations: an empirical study. Sustain For. 2022;14(5):2570.
47. Babu R, Bahuleyan B, Panchu P, Shilpa AV, Sreeja CK, Manjuran DJ. Effectiveness of self-paced and instructor-led online learning: a study among phase I medical students. J Clin Diagn Res. 2022;16(1)
48. Lai-Kwon J, Woodward-Kron R, Seignior D, Allen LM, McArthur G, Barrett M, et al. Qualitative evaluation of a multidisciplinary master of cancer sciences: impacts on graduates and influencing curricular factors. BMC Med Educ. 2024;
49. Razmerita L, Kirchner K. Collaboration and E-collaboration: a study of factors that influence perceived students' group performance. In: 2015 48th Hawaii international conference on system sciences. IEEE; 2015. p. 33–42.
50. Kok DL, Dushyanthen S, Peters G, Sapkaroski D, Barrett M, Sim J, et al. Virtual reality and augmented reality in radiation oncology education – a review and expert commentary. Tech Innov Patient Support Radiat Oncol. 2022;24:25–31.
51. Moore RL. The role of data analytics in education: possibilities and limitations. In: Responsible analytics and data mining in education. Routledge; 2018. p. 101–18.
52. Silén C, Wirell S, Kvist J, Nylander E, Smedby Ö. Advanced 3D visualization in student-centred medical education. Med Teach. 2008;30(5):e115–24.
53. Kumar S, Todd G. Effectiveness of online learning interventions on student engagement and academic performance amongst first-year students in allied health disciplines: a systematic review of the literature. Focus Health Prof Educ Multi-Prof J. 2022;23(3):36–55.
54. Jiang Y, Liu Q, Yu S, Ma J, Wu L. Exploring the continuous learning willingness under the risk of data breach in online learning system: a Fuzzy-Set QCA approach. In: 2022 International symposium on educational technology (ISET), vol. 2022. IEEE. p. 98–101.
55. Xhaferi B, Xhaferi G. Online learning benefits and challenges during the COVID 19-pandemic-students' perspective from SEEU. Seeu Rev. 2020;15(1):86–103.
56. Baranova K, Driman DK. Staying online in uncertain times: a Nationwide Canadian survey of pathology resident uses of and adaptations to online learning during COVID-19. Arch Pathol Lab Med. 2023;147(11):1333–9.
57. Fabito BS, Trillanes AO, Sarmiento JR. Barriers and challenges of computing students in an online learning environment: Insights from one private university in the Philippines. ArXiv Prepr ArXiv201202121. 2020
58. Jona CM, Sheen JA, O'Shea M. Benefits and challenges of an online CBT group, utilizing self-practice/self-reflection paradigm for psychology trainees. Train Educ Prof Psychol. 2022;
59. Aljaraideh Y. Massive open online learning (MOOC) benefits and challenges: a case study in Jordanian context. Int J Instr. 2019;12(4):65–78.
60. Simpson O. Student retention in distance education: are we failing our students? Open Learn J Open Distance E-Learn. 2013;28(2):105–19.
61. Boston W, Ice P, Burgess M. Assessing student retention in online learning environments: a longitudinal study. Online J Distance Learn Adm. 2012;15(2):1–6.
62. James R. Tertiary student attitudes to invigilated, online summative examinations. Int J Educ Technol High Educ. 2016;13:1–13.
63. Ghanbarzadeh R, Ghapanchi AH. Drivers of users' embracement of 3D digital educational spaces in higher education: a qualitative approach. Technol Knowl Learn. 2023;28(4):1707–44.
64. Buxton MJ. Problems in the economic appraisal of new health technology: the evaluation of heart transplants in the UK. Econ Apprais Health Technol Eur Community Oxf Oxf Med Publ. 1987:103–18.

65. De Oliveira M, Andrew Miles J, Asbridge. Modern medical schools curricula: necessary innovations and priorities for change. J Eval Clin Pract. 2023;
66. Klamen DL, Williams RG, Hingle S, Hingle S. Getting real: aligning the learning needs of clerkship students with the current clinical environment. Acad Med. 2019;94(1):53–8.
67. Paton M, Kuper A, Paradis E, Feilchenfeld Z, Whitehead C. Tackling the void: the importance of addressing absences in the field of health professions education research. Adv Health Sci Educ. 2021;26(1):5–18.
68. Salim SY, White J. Swimming in a tsunami of change. Adv Health Sci Educ. 2018;23(2):407–11.
69. Servant-Miklos VFC. A revolution in its own right: how Maastricht University reinvented problem-based learning. Health Prof Educ. 2019;5(4):283–93.
70. Whitehead C. Getting off the carousel: De-centring the curriculum in medical education. Perspect Med Educ. 2017;6(5):283–5.
71. Harden RM, Harden RM, Grant J, Buckley G, Hart IR. BEME Guide No. 1: best evidence medical education. Med Teach. 1999;21(6):553–62.
72. Norman GR. The birth and death of curricula. Adv Health Sci Educ. 2017;22(4):797–801.
73. Binks AP, LeClair RJ, Willey JM, Brenner JM, Pickering JD, Moore JS, et al. Changing medical education, overnight: the curricular response to COVID-19 of nine medical schools. Teach Learn Med. 2021;33(3):334–42.
74. Hertling SF, Back DA, Eckhart N, Kaiser M, Graul I. How far has the digitization of medical teaching progressed in times of COVID-19? A multinational survey among medical students and lecturers in German-speaking Central Europe. BMC Med Educ. 2022;22(1):387.
75. Young JQ, Van Merrienboer J, Durning S, Ten Cate O. Cognitive load theory: implications for medical education: AMEE guide No. 86. Med Teach. 2014;36(5):371–84.
76. Kok DL, Dushyanthen S, Giuliani M, Garda AE, Golden DW. Chapter 106 - education to translate research into practice. In: Eltorai AEM, Bakal JA, Kim DW, Wazer DE, editors. Translational radiation oncology [Internet]. Academic Press. p. 647–52. 2023 [cited 2024 May 25]. (Handbook for Designing and Conducting Clinical and Translational Research). Available from: https://www.sciencedirect.com/science/article/pii/B9780323884235001047.
77. Johnstone A, El-banna H. Capacities, demands and processes—a predictive model for science education. Educ Chem. 1986:23.
78. Opdenacker C, Fierens H, Brabant HV, Sevenants J, Spruyt J, Slootmaekers PJ, et al. Academic performance in solving chemistry problems related to student working memory capacity. Int J Sci Educ. 1990;12(2):177–85.
79. Allan Paivio, Paivio A. Mental representations: A dual coding approach. 1986
80. Cuevas J, Dawson BL. A test of two alternative cognitive processing models: learning styles and dual coding. Theory Res Educ. 2018;16(1):40–64.
81. Mayer RE, Mayer RE, Moreno R, Moreno R. Nine ways to reduce cognitive load in multimedia learning. Educ Psychol. 2003;38(1):43–52.
82. Krumm IR, Miles MC, Clay A, Carlos Ii WG, Adamson R. Making effective educational videos for clinical teaching. Chest. 2022;161(3):764–72.
83. Larochelle M, Bednarz N, Garrison JW. Constructivism and education. Cambridge University Press; 1998. 332 p
84. Bandura A, Walters RH. Social learning theory, vol. 1. Englewood cliffs Prentice Hall; 1977.
85. Goldie JGS. Connectivism: a knowledge learning theory for the digital age? Med Teach. 2016;38(10):1064–9.
86. Kolb DA. Experiential learning: experience as the source of learning and development. FT Press; 2014.
87. Knowles MS. Andragogy, not pedagogy. 1968.
88. Hanson A. The search for a separate theory of adult learning: does anyone really need andragogy? In: Boundaries of adult learning. Routledge; 1996.

89. Bencherki N. Actor–network theory. In: The international encyclopedia of organizational communication [Internet]. Wiley. p. 1–13. 2017 [cited 2024 May 27]. Available from: https://onlinelibrary.wiley.com. https://doi.org/10.1002/9781118955567.wbieoc002.
90. Mezirow J. A transformation theory of adult learning. In: Adult education research annual conference proceedings [Internet]. ERIC; 1993 [cited 2024 Jun 17]. p. 141–6. Available from: https://files.eric.ed.gov/fulltext/ED357160.pdf#page=153

Chapter 2
Designing Effective, Online Health Professional Curricula

David L. Kok, Michelle Barrett, Sathana Dushyanthen, and David Seignior

Abstract Online education has become increasingly available, sophisticated, and affordable in the post COVID-19 era. In addition, learner appetite and expectation for online learning experiences have increased exponentially in health professional education (HPE). As such, health professional educators should be considering in what ways their curricula can better incorporate online techniques and how to do this in a way that authentically leverages the natural strengths of the new medium rather than simply porting learning activities that were designed for face-to-face settings into an online medium.

This chapter outlines how health professional educators can go about (re)designing health education curricula to be fit-for-purpose for online education. A ground-up method of curriculum development is advocated and described using Kern's 6-step model of curriculum development, with a particular focus on the implementation stage which has numerous specific aspects that are unique to online curriculum design. In addition, we introduce core pedagogical considerations in online curriculum design including modularity, sequencing of learning activities and use of the Technological, Pedagogical, Content Knowledge (TPACK) framework.

The chapter then concludes by outlining the practicalities of online curriculum development and describing some of the tips and tricks that educators should know to successfully navigate this process.

D. L. Kok (✉)
Peter MacCallum Cancer Centre, Melbourne, VIC, Australia

University of Melbourne, Melbourne, VIC, Australia

Monash University, Melbourne, VIC, Australia
e-mail: dkok@unimelb.edu.au

M. Barrett
Victorian Comprehensive Cancer Centre, Melbourne, VIC, Australia

S. Dushyanthen · D. Seignior
University of Melbourne, Melbourne, VIC, Australia

© The Author(s), under exclusive license to Springer Nature Switzerland AG 2025
D. L. Kok et al. (eds.), *Best Practices in Online Education*, IAMSE Manuals,
https://doi.org/10.1007/978-3-031-90349-6_2

Key Points

- Health professional educators should be proactively incorporating online education into their formal curricula and leveraging the natural benefits of the medium.
- Curricular design (and re-design) is best approached in a systematic, ground-up method.
- The 6-step model of curriculum development, as originally described by Kern, is an effective framework for scaffolding online design and re-design processes.
- The 6-steps are: (1) problem identification and general needs assessment; (2) targeted needs assessment; (3) goals and objectives; (4) educational strategies; (5) implementation; (6) evaluation, feedback and continuous improvement.
- The implementation phase is especially extended in online education as the design and building of learning experiences is relatively complex. It is worth considering this stage in 3 sub-phases: A) Team assembly; B) Designing the Curriculum; C) Delivery/rollout of the curriculum.
- Core pedagogical considerations in online learning include the 'Technology, Pedagogy and Content Knowledge' (TPACK) framework, modularity, and sequencing of activities.

2.1 Introduction: The Importance of Keeping Health Professional Curricula Current

While there are many aspects which must be considered when creating an educational program, including its objectives, pedagogical factors, the delivery context, the variety of learning tools available, and methods of assessment- ultimately, they must fit together to create a unified, coherent teaching package. The overarching structure that encompasses all of these elements is the curriculum.

There continues to be some variation in the definition of 'curriculum,' even among medical education experts [1]. Hence, for clarity, throughout this chapter and this manual, the following definition is used.

> *Curriculum – A learning experience or group of learning experiences that comprises a discrete educational program or package.*

And the following curricula subtypes are defined as follows:

> *Formal curriculum – The planned, formally documented, and intentional learning experience(s) that together can be identified as a discrete educational program or package.*

> *Hidden curriculum* – *The undocumented, often unintentional, learning experiences that occur incidentally within a discrete program or package.*

The importance of a quality formal curriculum is obvious. It is through well-designed formal curricula that we can provide quality HPE [2, 3]. And it is through quality HPE, that we can create a proficient, effective healthcare workforce that delivers excellent patient outcomes [4].

But what comprises a 'quality' curriculum?

The quality of an educational program may be best thought of as one which is fit-for-purpose.

Currently, there is no consensus around the criteria that determine whether a curriculum remains fit for purpose [5]. However, accreditation standards [6, 7] and expert opinion [8, 9] do converge on a few major criteria:

1. that the curriculum is tailored to the needs of the educational audience.
2. that the knowledge and skills imparted within the curriculum are up to date.
3. that the curriculum is effective and efficient in the transmission of knowledge/skills to its learners, i.e., It utilizes effective pedagogical design principles.

However, each of these measured factors is not static. In fact, they are constantly evolving. Therefore, for a curriculum to remain fit for purpose, it must evolve as well or run the risk of becoming outdated. Outdated curricula can impact eventual healthcare delivery. In particular, there is a risk that the knowledge and/or skills imparted to the students in the program may no longer be clinically relevant [10] (e.g., it may not include new classes of drugs that have gone to market after the curriculum was initially designed. Or new medical equipment may have been released, making prior models obsolete).

From a delivery standpoint, recent major technological advances, including Wi-Fi, smartphones, virtual reality, cloud-based computing, and social media, [11] have ushered in an era characterized by the ubiquity of technology and, specifically, *the internet* in all aspects of daily life [12, 13]. In line with this, it has also introduced a range of new, engaging, and flexible learning experiences that were previously impossible. Thus, it is incumbent upon educators to actively consider how online techniques could be incorporated into our teaching practices through a process of curriculum design/redesign and to do this in the most effective way possible.

Just like in traditional education - there is no set recipe for curriculum success in the online domain. The chosen curriculum structure must take into consideration the intended audience, context, purpose, and learning outcomes of the program. When one considers each of these factors, one can then purposefully decide which pedagogical options are most likely to meet the needs of their learners and give the best chance to design a fit-for-purpose learning activity. In addition, it should be noted that in any given context many potential curricula may be equally effective in achieving the desired learning outcomes – there is not necessarily one 'correct' solution.

Conversely, though, there will be suboptimal solutions. Thus, educators should strive to engage in a meaningful design process that matches educational theory with the needs of their learners.

2.2 Taking a Systematic Approach to Curricular Design and Redesign

While there is a constant need for quality improvement processes to 'fine tune' a learning program, implementing online education is a cardinal change in both pedagogy and delivery platforms. To design a curriculum in such a way that genuinely leverages the inherent strengths and weaknesses of the new technique typically requires a fundamental reform of the learning experience.

This was well demonstrated during COVID-19 period when mandatory change to online delivery occurred in tertiary HPE programs worldwide. Due to the unexpected nature of this change, and the speed which it needed to be implemented, most implementations of online education in this period were simplistic at best and, in most cases, a direct transposition of an existing curriculum into the online space through digital delivery means. For instance, what had traditionally been in-person lectures were then recorded for online consumption or delivered over Zoom, but often not changing the overall timing (e.g., 1-h), format (e.g., PowerPoint slides and teacher) or content.

Unsurprisingly, programs that adopted this simplistic approach were not always well-received by learners, with many reports of poorer student engagement, worse student experience ratings, and a desire (in some settings) to return to original learning formats as soon as local regulations allowed it [14]. On the other hand, programs that undertook bespoke design processes that leveraged the natural strengths of online learning were often received more favourably [15].

With this in mind, we advocate a 'ground up' approach to online curriculum design – in effect thinking as if one was constructing a new curriculum, even if a prior curriculum does exist. Attempting to retain elements from an existing program and retrofitting them into a new online structure often result in incongruity due to those elements having been removed from the wider context in which they were originally designed for. One can consider the analogy of a builder performing a knockdown and rebuild of an old house rather than the more difficult task of maintaining one or two rooms and incorporating them into a new structure. This view is also reflected when one looks at published experiences of curricula renewal; in nearly all cases where a renewal involved the incorporation of a new underlying pedagogy, the 'curricula renewal' was, in effect, de novo, with minimal (if any) discussion of how prior structures were retained into the new program.

While this task may seem complex and overwhelming, it need not be. A systematic approach helps to break this process down into feasible individual steps. We herein describe a workflow that is divided into two major aspects – firstly, several core online design principles that should be applied longitudinally across all aspects of an online curriculum, and secondly, a step-by-step process of curriculum design that is universal to all HPE curricula. When used in conjunction, these provide an effective scaffold for online HPE design.

It is important to emphasize that these principles are applicable for use in curricula of any size, ranging from as small as a simple 2 h learning module to a multi-year interconnected degree program. This is relevant as this manual has deliberately taken a broad view of online HPE, understanding that curricula can (and should) be of all types, shapes, and sizes.

2.3 Core Online Curriculum Design Considerations

When designing an online curriculum, there are some specific pedagogical considerations that should be universal to all programs. These are outlined here.

2.3.1 Technological, Pedagogical, Content Knowledge (TPACK) Framework

The TPACK model can be used as a way of framing how we think about modern educational design [16, 17]. It is best depicted as a Venn diagram (Fig. 2.1) that highlights three major domains of knowledge that teachers must utilise in the design of learning experiences:

- Content knowledge – the instructor's knowledge about the relevant subject matter.
- Pedagogical knowledge – the instructor's knowledge of instructional processes and theories of learning.
- Technological knowledge – the instructor's knowledge of the various technologies that can be used for teaching and how to apply them.

The TPACK model highlights how educational design relies on knowledge of all three of these areas, and it is only through the intersection of all three of these that optimal design can be applied. This is a challenge for modern educators, as staying up to date in even just one of these domains may be difficult. That said, educators may find it reassuring to know that it is not necessary (or expected) for any single individual to have expert-level knowledge of each of these domains. In fact, to design optimal learning experiences inherently requires large and diverse teams that can integrate the skills of many individuals to deliver the end-product. What is required, however, is an understanding of the broad principles across all three domains to be able to create a quality, fit-for-purpose curriculum 'blueprint'. This

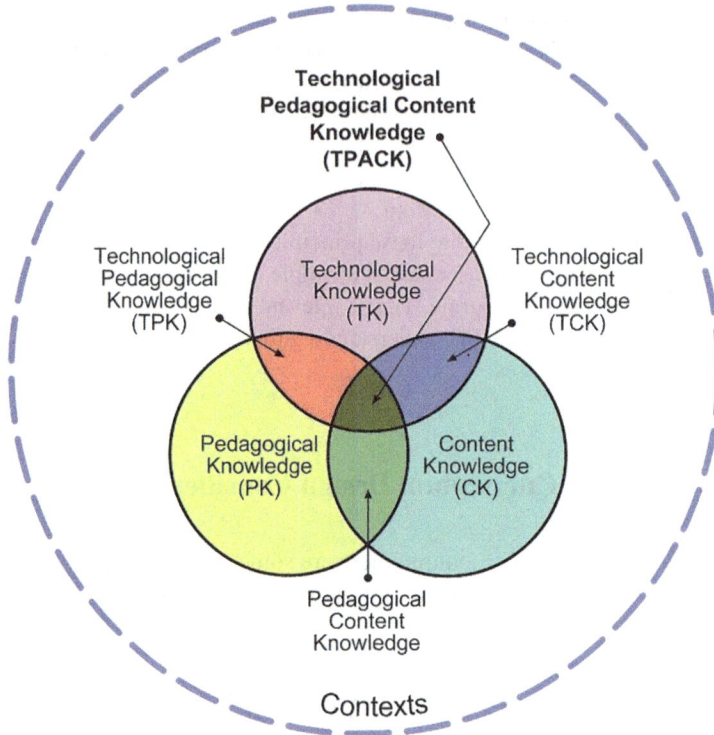

Fig. 2.1 The Technological, Pedagogical, Content Knowledge (TPACK) framework (from Koehler and Mishra [16]) (Reproduced by permission of the publisher, © 2012 by tpack.org)

blueprint can then be used to guide the efforts of team members with specialized skillets to work together synergistically in the construction and delivery of the curriculum.

This manual aims to give an educator a solid understanding of the basic principles across the *technological* and *pedagogical* domains to be able to make sound design decisions in a curriculum design process. For instance, we will discuss principles of gamification and how to best utilize it (in Chap. 4). Ultimately, the skill set we are aiming to foster is analogous to the chief designer of an aircraft, who does not necessarily know the details of how to build a jet engine, but does know their capabilities and also knows how and when to bring a jet-engineer onto their team to fulfil that specific need.

2.3.2 Modularity and Self-Pacing of the Curriculum

A specific educational strategy that is well-suited to online education is modularity and self-pacing of the curriculum [18, 19]. Modularity is where one designs learning experiences into discrete, coherent components that are self-contained and achieve specific learning objectives within themselves. (In the school education context, this is sometimes referred to as 'chunking'). Thus, each module can potentially be delivered individually without being reliant on prior or later learning tasks.

This gives flexibility across multiple domains:

- Firstly, it allows flexibility of the overall curriculum design. Inherently, all learners enter a program with different backgrounds and have different goals they are aiming to achieve. Modularity allows learners to assemble a curriculum that accounts for these individual differences, retaining pre-defined core elements alongside additional elective modules. Thus, ensuring learning material is relevant to everyone's needs.
- Modularity allows regular revisitation of learning material – a form of self-pacing and an important method of memory consolidation.
- Modularity allows self-pacing at a macro level through the ability to start and stop learning based on convenience and/or memory saturation. This is particularly important for health professionals and health profession students who are frequently time-poor [20] and may only have short intervals in their routine to undertake learning activities

Asynchronous, self-paced, online delivery is an excellent application of modularity and hence is widely used in online education. It utilizes the natural strengths of the medium, removing the traditional educational limitation of being forced to move at a fixed speed that is determined by instructors or classmates.

> **Tip:** When creating a modular curriculum, there is no set 'size' for the modules/learning activities. This is highly dependent on the type and context of the learning program you are creating. However, as a rule of thumb, a module should revolve around a core learning outcome within the curriculum which can, therefore, be learnt as a standalone item. It is also helpful if the module can be completed in a single sitting, as health professionals may not have the ability to return to the material quickly and may thus experience significant cognitive loss in the interim.

2.3.3 Sequencing of Activities

Even motivated learners have finite concentration spans. Fatigue and inattention builds quickly, particularly in the online context [21] where others apps (such as social media) are only a single click away. Data from online educational videos demonstrate that there is a sharp drop-off in video viewership after only 6–7 min of viewing [22, 23].

Therefore, one could characterize online education programs as existing in a constant state of competition with other distractors. One way of maintaining learners' attention and engagement is by a method wherein the curriculum is regularly moving between a diverse range of educational formats (e.g. between video, text and interactive content). Not only does this help to sustain the leaner's engagement with the material, it is also useful to prevent information through multiple 'lenses', therefore increasing the likelihood of successful long-term retention (this is sometimes referred to as using 'multiple means of representation' to aid learning [24]).

> **Tip:** Aim to move between delivery formats at durations of approximately 5–10 min. This falls below the standard threshold for inattention in online learning.

Chapter 4 describes different learning formats and the relevant digital learning tools that one can use online in a more detailed discussion.

2.4 Kern's Curriculum Development Model

The most widely known and utilised model for curriculum development in HPE is the six-step model that was first described by Kern in 1998. Originally proposed as a framework for the design of entry-to-practice medical curricula, it has since gained widespread popularity throughout all HPE, and subsequent editions have expanded on its basic principles to be more generalisable. Although not specific for design of online curricula, it remains an effective model for broadly scaffolding a curricular design process. We outline each of the steps in relation to online curriculum design but have especially focused on the implementation stage, as this stage is markedly different in online education compared to traditional formats. Therefore, we have expanded and divided Implementation into three sub-phases – 'Team Assembly', 'Designing the Curriculum' and 'Delivery/Rollout of the Curriculum'.

The six steps are depicted in Fig. 2.2.

2.4.1 Problem Identification and General Needs Assessment

This involves the identification of the educational need, or gap, that requires addressing. This initial identification is performed at an extremely broad level and does not yet relate to the individual needs of your specific, intended audience.

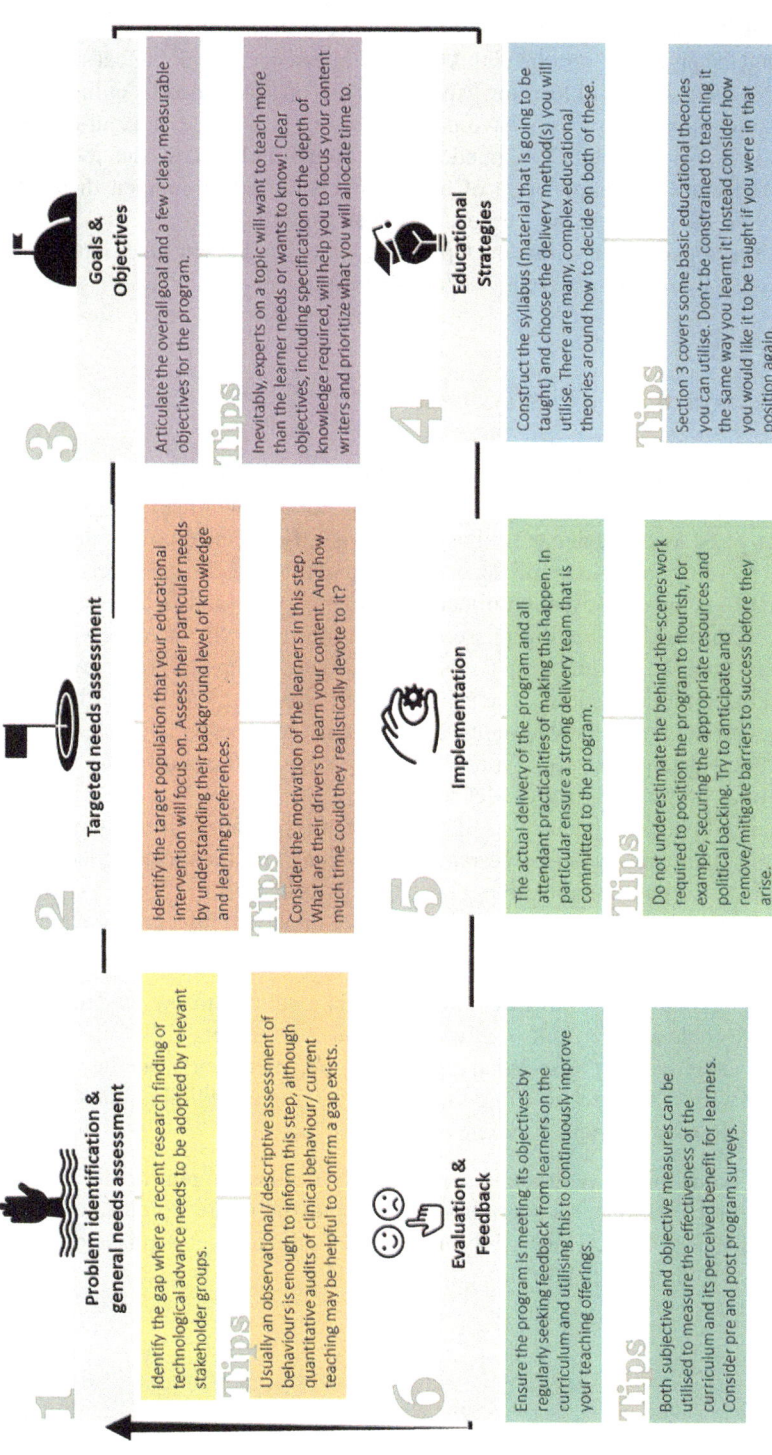

Fig. 2.2 Kern's curriculum development model with tips for educators (from Kok et al. [25])

A broad identification of the need for online education has been articulated in Chap. 1 and the preceding section of this Chapter. In essence, technological advances have enabled a new class of learning experiences that are facilitated by online delivery. These learning experiences have the potential to be flexible, student-centred, high-yield, non-geographically bounded, and highly tailored to the individual learner. Therefore, the application of online education can strengthen these elements and produce more fit-for-purpose HPE learning programs.

Given the above, curriculum developers need not spend much time on this step and can move to the more substantive steps that follow.

2.4.2 Targeted Needs Assessment

Once one has agreed on the general need, educators must then look at their own specific context and assess the needs of that particular group of learners.

This targeted assessment can be thought of as a self-contained project that could be tasked to a curriculum-committee, or subgroup of this. An effective needs assessment comprises two phases: an information-gathering phase and an analysis phase.

In the information-gathering phase, utilize a tool that will effectively sample your learner cohort. Common methods include focus groups, surveys, review of prior feedback, and interviews. The principles of performing this type of information gathering are not specific to online education and thus beyond the scope of this manual. For a detailed description of this we recommend the text by Stufflebeam [26] or, for a shorter read, that of McCawley [27].

The second phase is the analysis of the gathered information. Identify the common themes that exist, what is the range of opinions, are there clear educational gaps evident, and how can the different needs be prioritised?

In the online HPE setting, it is particularly important to understand questions around:

- Existing technological infrastructure - what is available to the students, how knowledgeable are they in its use, what bottlenecks exist, etc.
- Learner experience factors – What types of learning experiences are they looking for, and what is their relative importance? For example, flexibility, interactivity, individual/group learning, time capacity, etc.

This process can take several months, particularly if it is a large program and one wants to source opinions from current learners, potential future learners, and those of program stakeholders. Thus, a 3–6-month time frame for this step is appropriate for programs at the degree level.

2.4.3 Goals and Objectives

With a clear understanding of the needs of the learners, one can then use this information to begin articulating the goals and objectives of the new curriculum.

In an educational sense, goals are typically broad, describing an overall aim of the program that can be aspirational. An objective is much more specific and should be measurable.

An example may be:

- The goal is 'for social work students undertaking this program to develop the skills, knowledge and attitudes to safely and effectively navigate emotionally charged conversations in the course of their work '
- A learning objective within this program could be 'that students demonstrate three conversational de-escalation techniques in a simulated environment.'

This step is also when key decisions should be made around the size and scope of the project being undertaken. Resourcing will have a key influence on this, and thus, this is also the stage when one should begin sourcing the resources required for the educational project.

This may lead to an iterative process where the goal and scope of the project are refined to meet the available resourcing and vice versa until a feasible and practical balance between the two is met. Thus, the time taken to solidify these can vary quite markedly depending on the number of revisions and the number of executive layers this needs to go through to be 'signed off.' 2–4 months is a reasonable allocation for a degree-level course.

The process of writing learning objectives has a deep literature base of its own, but for those wishing to explore this process, we suggest reviewing the primer written by Chatterjee [28] for further guidance on this topic.

2.4.4 Educational Strategies

Educators can then begin the process of choosing the educational strategies that are aligned to the needs of your cohort, and the goals and objectives of the program.

We suggest creation of a table that itemizes the key needs/issues of the cohort. Then, identify the appropriate learning theories and pedagogical principles that can address these (these were discussed in Chap. 1). Then, having considered your context/resourcing (as described in Chap. 3), identify the appropriate learning tools that you will use to respond to these (detailed in Chap. 4).

In Table 2.1 we provide a real-life example of how this process was performed and subsequently implemented.

2.4.5 Implementation – Phase A: Team Assembly (Including Online Education Skillsets)

Kern's original publication referred to the fifth stage of curriculum design simply as 'implementation'. Here we have subdivided these further into three substages - 'team assembly', 'design' and the 'delivery' of the curriculum. In the online setting each of these phases is sizable and hence worthy of discussion in its own right.

Table 2.1 Example of how pedagogical strategies were mapped to address the specific needs of cancer professionals in an online degree in cancer sciences (Excerpt from Lai Kwon et al. [29])

Key issue	Pedagogy	Solution
Diverse geographic location of cohort	• Online delivery method	• Wholly online course, accessible from any device and designed to be responsive.
Heterogeneity of cohort in terms of discipline and level of experience	• Flexibility of curriculum design • High touch supervision	• Flexible format with core subjects and electives • Nested award format • Low bar to entry with a stepwise approach to resource levelling • Regular interaction and live webinars with subject tutors • Practical toolkits
Time poor participants with competing priorities and distractions	• Cognitive load theory • Cognitive theory of multimedia learning • Visual information design theory	• Present material in succinct, 'chunked' packages • Infographics • Screen-based learning methods • Interactivity and gamification • Augmented/visual reality
Complexity of oncological material	• Cognitive load theory • Cognitive theory of multimedia learning	• Tailored choice of delivery medium to suit individual lesson • Infographics • Bespoke educational videos allowing dynamic on-screen drawing, eye contact, purposeful visual cuing • Branching scenarios to promote experiential learning • Gamification to allow practice, reinforcement, and review of key concepts

(continued)

Table 2.1 (continued)

Key issue	Pedagogy	Solution
Need for knowledge and skills applicable to practice	• Applied learning design • Industry-based and sector-leading teaching team • Reproduction of real tasks as assessment tasks	• Patient and multidisciplinary-focused case studies • Expert interviews • Panel discussions • Mock multidisciplinary meetings to replicate real-world interactions • Assessments promoting application of learnings to the real-world context
Need to promote multidisciplinary learning	• All students come with prior knowledge and experience allowing them to contribute meaningfully to the course • Interprofessionality and interprofessional education	• Discussion boards to facilitate learning from peers • Group work • Clinical role plays
Integration of the lived experience of consumers throughout the curriculum design and delivery	• Consumers as educators • Simulation • Co-design • Integrating lived experience in research	• Expert consumer interviews and reflections • Consumers as expert panellists • Simulated clinician/patient scenarios • Consumers as research capstone supervisors to ensure consumer inclusion in research design

The first step of this implementation step is the assembly of a proficient curriculum design team. The size of this will be dependent upon the learning program being designed, and the resources available. However, in general, teams required for building online programs can be quite large, and there are numerous roles and skillsets where are not directly analogous to traditional curricula, hence it is important to have weighed each of these prior to commencing the design and ensuring there are individuals which possess these skillsets in your team.

The requisite skillsets can be broadly grouped into several key categories, these are: Educational leadership (Fig. 2.3), Online teaching and facilitation (Fig. 2.4), Instructional design (Fig. 2.5), Content creation (Fig. 2.6), Educational technology and video production (Fig. 2.7), and Evaluation and education research (Fig. 2.8).

This is a long list, and reflective of how educational curricula have evolved over time. Once again, it is worthwhile noting that although some select individuals may possess more than one of these skillsets, as online education becomes increasingly advanced, it is becoming harder and harder for any educator to maintain multiple proficiencies at a high level and so a team of individuals representing these skillsets is the best way of accounting for these.

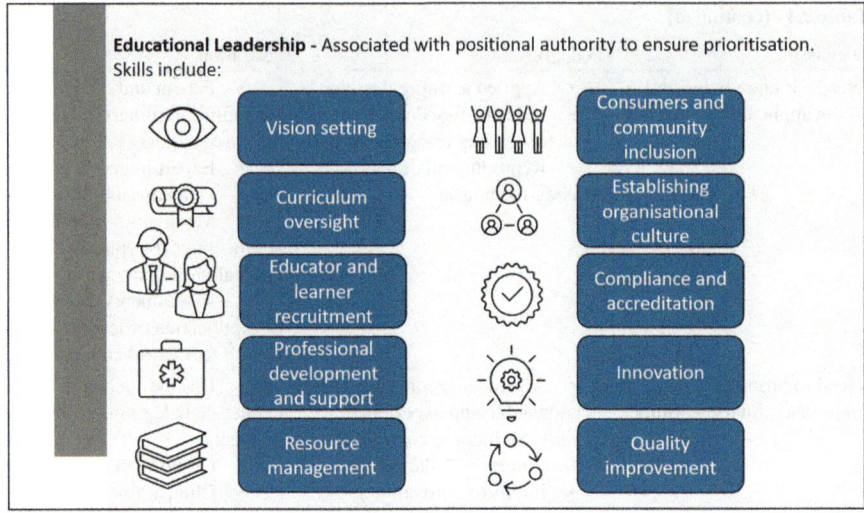

Fig. 2.3 Educational Leadership skills required in online education

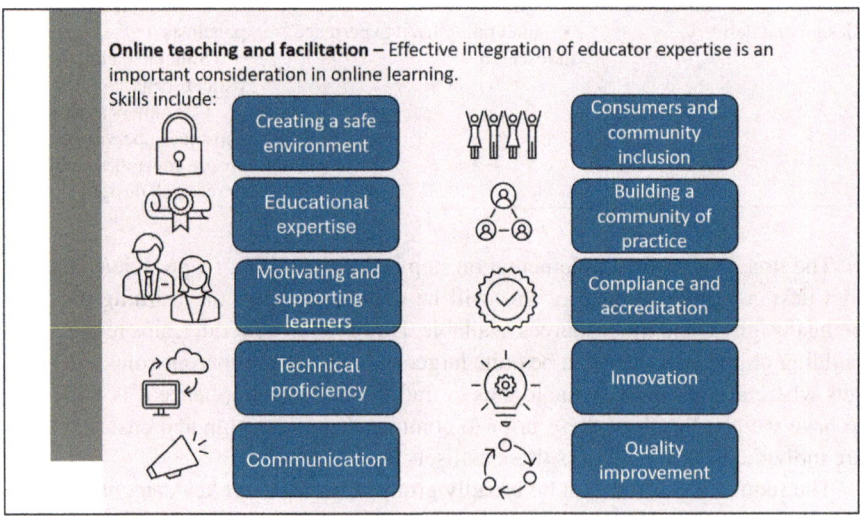

Fig. 2.4 Online teaching and facilitation skills required in online education

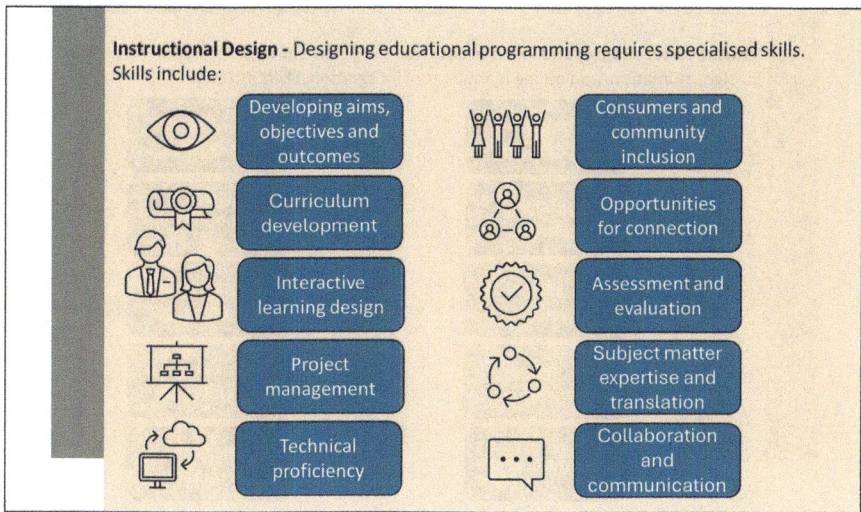

Fig. 2.5 Instructional Design skills required in online education

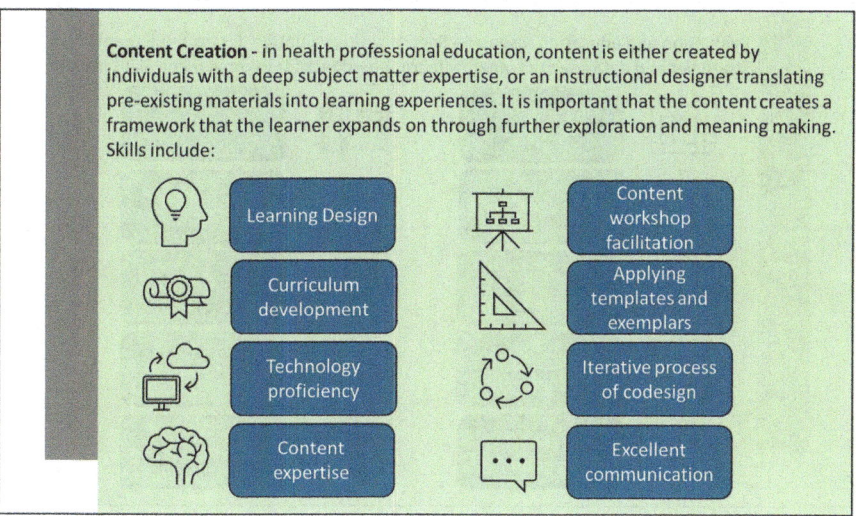

Fig. 2.6 Content Creation skills required in online education

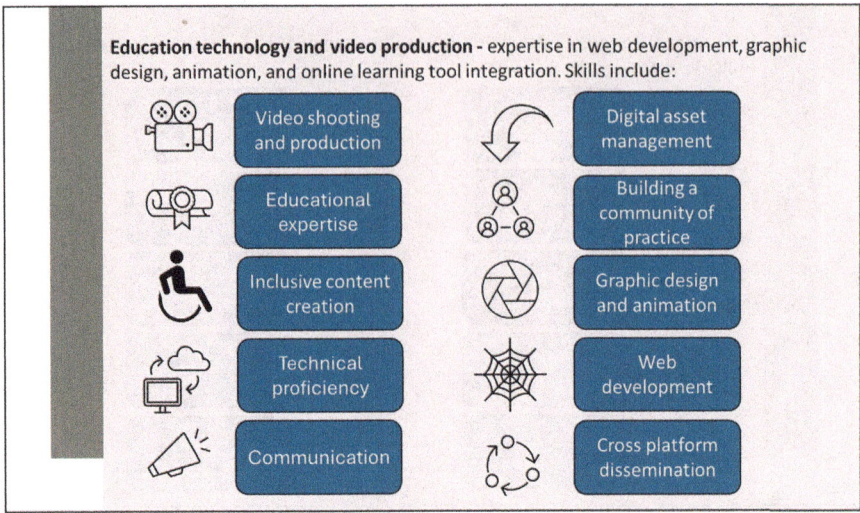

Fig. 2.7 Educational technology and video production skills required in online education

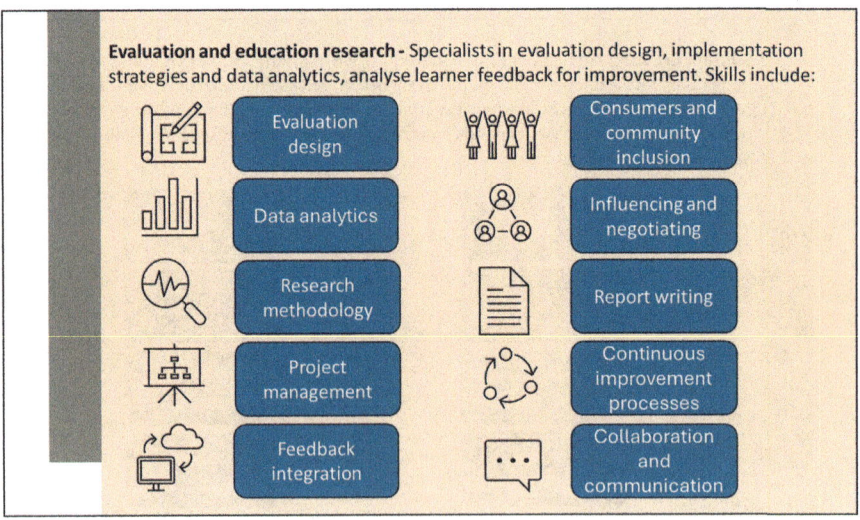

Fig. 2.8 Evaluation and education research skills required in online education

> **Tip:** To efficiently and effectively develop a curriculum is no small task. When assembling a core team to tackle this, it requires a combination of educational knowledge, proven experience, and (perhaps most important of all) people who are enthusiastic about the change with a can-do attitude. Refrain from making the team too big; large committees are unwieldy and more likely to dilute responsibility so that everybody believes 'someone else will do the hard work.' As such, it is the educators who are willing to do the heavy lifting of writing and creating educational products that should be the engine of a curricular design team.

2.4.6 Implementation – Phase B: Designing the Curriculum

Once one has established the team, the actual work of development can begin.

The individual components of the curriculum should each be considered. These are:

- **The learning context**

    Online learning contexts and how they influence curricular design are discussed in Chap. 3.

- **Goals/Intended learning outcomes**

    'Learning outcomes' describe the intended outcome from a curriculum or program, which is different to 'learning objectives' which describe what a learner should have achieved at the end of an individual learning experience. Often, they are matched to the goals of the program to provide yardsticks that ensure that the aims of the program are being met. The design of intended learning outcomes is no different in the online setting from any other educational setting and, hence, is not covered in this manual. However, for those looking for a quick guide to writing these, we suggest reviewing the guide by Popenici [30].

- **Curricular structure**

    Curricular structure is not specific to the online domain and is not explored in detail in this book. That being said, the 'core and special study modules' principle described by Harden in 2009 [31] is now a well-recognized and highly effective structure to consider as a baseline. In addition, the following section in this chapter discusses the principle of modularity of the curriculum and how this can be utilised, given it is a natural strength of online curricula.

- **Learning activities**

    Online learning has a variety of unique learning tools that can be used to create learning activities. These are discussed in Chap. 4.

- **Teaching and facilitation techniques**

    Teaching and facilitation in the online arena are technically and qualitatively different from face-to-face teaching. These differences and methods to excel in the online environment are discussed in Chap. 5.

It is important to ensure that each component of the curriculum work together seamlessly together to produce a single, unified learning experience. Constructive alignment can be used to do this [32], which contends that all features of a program (the structure, activities, assessments, and teaching techniques) need to be aligned directly to intended learning outcomes. This is commonly done by defining the learning outcomes first and then constructing the other components in reference to these. While constructive alignment may seem obvious, it is not uncommon for inexperienced educators to begin by designing learning experiences first and then crafting learning objectives afterward, a method which frequently leads to a mismatch between the two.

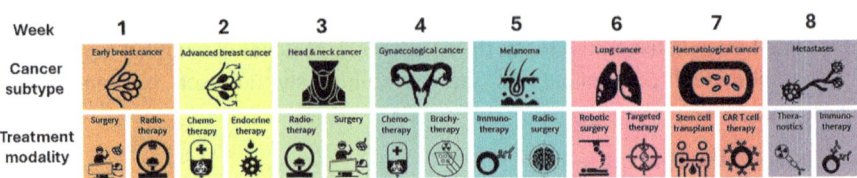

Each week we will discuss a different type of cancer and the principles of two different treatment modalities that are pertinent to that cancer type. Where a treatment modality is revisited more than once, more advanced concepts will be introduced each time.

Fig. 2.9 Example of a subject roadmap for a cancer science subject

Another useful method, that can be used alongside constructive alignment, is the creation of a clear overarching 'roadmap' of the different modules within a curriculum. This assists both educators and learners to quickly identifying where essential information lies within these and helps to ensure that there is a logical, and iterative learning experience that builds throughout the curriculum [33] (see Fig. 2.9 **for an example**). Furthermore, it can help orientate learners, so they know where they are in their journeys (and potentially select learning modules based on their prior levels of knowledge).

Given the complexity of the design phase, educators should be prepared for this to be the most time-consuming aspect of any curricular reform project. A year or more in this design phase would be a reasonable expectation for a degree-level program.

2.4.7 Implementation – Phase C: Delivery/Rollout of the New Curriculum

The actual rollout of a new curriculum is most likely to be successful if one has a structured plan for the process. Adequate preparation, an orderly roll-out timeline (including redundancies to account for when things do not go according to plan), and adequately preparing both the educators and learners for the changes that are about to occur will all smooth the actual process of implementation.

It is worth noting that online education also provides an unusual opportunity for detailed beta-testing and review of learning experiences before being released for student consumption. Beta-testers may comprise current or former students, academic staff members or even professionally hired testers. Because many online experiences are asynchronous by nature, this means there may be the ability to pass through multiple rounds of review before a proper 'hard launch.'

2.4.8 Evaluation, Feedback and Continuous Improvement

All educational programs should have evaluation and feedback processes to continuously assess their success at meeting their goal and objectives. This also provides information that can be used iteratively for continuous quality improvement of a curricula, a common requirement of many HPE accreditation bodies [34, 35].

Practice Point Despite the important role of evaluation in the curriculum development and review process, there remains a scarcity of widely used, validated instruments for this purpose. This was identified as a concern as far back as 2003 [36] and still remained the case in 2015 when Schiekirka et al. performed an extensive review of published curricular evaluation tools [37]. They identified only a single English instrument that assessed both curricular structures and processes – the Medical Student Experience Question (MedSEQ) [38], which was subsequently validated by Huang in 2023 [39]. As such we suggest this tool is used as a starting point for designing a curriculum evaluation, noting the following caveats:

- MedSEQ is a student-survey based evaluation. Full curricular evaluation benefits from the input of a wide-range of views, including those of faculty and other program stakeholders [40]. Adaptations of the survey to source these opinions is worth consideration.
- Surveys come with the risk of self-reporting bias. (This is where subjects may report things that they believe you want to hear, or reflects themselves in a more positive light [41]). Objectively measurable features may be worth capturing as part of a program evaluation (for instance, examination performance).
- Both quantitative and qualitative data are beneficial in evaluations. Qualitative data allows for a more in-depth and nuanced understanding of views and can also link specific aspects of a curriculum to effects, something quantitative data alone cannot [15].
- The impacts of a learning program may not be seen immediately after program delivery and it is beneficial to perform long-term evaluations after time has passed [42].

2.5 Curriculum Development Timelines

Developing a curriculum is a lengthy process and frequently underestimated by those taking on the task. In addition, the time taken can vary widely from program to program, as it is heavily influenced by factors such as the size of the curriculum, the extent of changes being made, the number of faculty involved in the process, and the financial resourcing available. In addition, there are often external fixed factors that a development team must attempt to meet – for instance, the almost immediate need for curriculum renewal in COVID-19 [43], or to meet an accreditation-mandated timeline [44]. When working to such fixed timelines, surprisingly fast curriculum transitions are possible, with case studies describing renewals of entire 4-year curricula in under 12 months [43, 45].

However, more typically, a whole degree transformation can take a number of years [29, 46–48], and we suggest (assuming appropriate resourcing) that 2–3 years is a reasonable timeframe. Timelines for smaller programs, for example, those at a subject or lesson level, can be estimated proportionate to their overall length using similar principles noted above. However, it should be noted that in the online domain, certain development aspects require set time periods, regardless of size. For example, an animated video would often have an expected production time of no less than 6–8 weeks due to the high level of preparation and editing involved [49].

2.6 An Applied Example of End-to-End Online Curricula Design

In 2018 a cancer-specific, multidisciplinary, wholly online degree was developed by members of our team. Kern's curriculum development framework was used to establish this, as detailed in Table 2.2.

2.7 Practicalities of Delivering Your Curriculum Online

Although the focus of this manual is on online educational factors that are directly relevant to academic teaching staff, a brief discussion of online technical infrastructure is included here as a basic understanding of these is important for all educators, even if many of the decisions around this are likely to be made at an institutional/executive level rather than by teaching staff. These choices also have a direct impact on what online educational methods can or cannot be utilized in a program.

2.7.1 *Hosting Your Curriculum Online*

In face-to-face learning programs, a key consideration is where the learning activities will be conducted - is it in a hospital, university, or other institution, and where is that located?

Online programs do not require considerations around the physical locale, but instead require a consideration of what is referred to as the *web hosting location*.

In its simplest terms, a web host is a service that stores your content online and makes it accessible to other internet users. It consists of a *server*, which is a computer that is constantly connected to the internet and has all your educational data loaded onto it. When another user connects to the internet and types the website

Table 2.2 Example of using Kern's Six-Step Approach in the Design of the University of Melbourne Master of Cancer Science Curriculum (From Lai Kwon et al. [29])

Steps	Approach in the masters of cancer sciences
1. *Problem identification and general needs assessment*	• Stakeholder engagement e.g. within the Victorian Comprehensive Cancer Centre (VCCC) Alliance, University of Melbourne • Board-level advice on educational landscape and need for masters course
2. *Targeted needs assessment*	• Market analysis to identify needs within the Australian and international oncology workforce by an external consulting firm
3. *Goals and objectives*	• Identification of subject, course and aggregate course-level learning outcomes
4. *Educational strategies*	• Central coordinating team of educational and academic experts to ensure a cohesive curriculum and consistency of vision • Formation of multidisciplinary expert working parties for each of the 10 cancer-specific subjects • Mapping of learning outcomes to course content and assessment tasks • Creation of course content using the seven principles of online learning and relevant pedagogical theories
5. *Implementation*	• Course delivered in 2019 • Multi-tiered promotional campaigninternal: University of Melbourne & the 10 VCCC Alliance Organisations external: Web (with search engine optimization-SEO), social media, conferences, traditional media

6. *Evaluation*	• Formation of a preliminary evaluation framework
	• Quantitative evaluation methods:
	  – University of Melbourne Student experience surveys conducted every 6 months during course participation
	  – Customised master of cancer sciences survey conducted 1-year post-graduation
	• Qualitative evaluation methods:
	  – Qualitative study to assess impact on career trajectory and professional practice (in progress)
	• Planned refresh of course content to incorporating student feedback and ongoing developments in the cancer sphere (each subject has a yearly minor refresh and triennial major refresh)

address into their browser, what they are in effect doing is sending a request to your server for the information stored within. The server then passes the data back to requester so they can view it. Servers are therefore the hardware on which your learning program is ultimately located. This is the same method by which all web pages and websites on the internet are stored.

There are two major ways to host an online educational resource. Many major academic institutions and hospitals have their own servers which are maintained and supported by their information technology teams. The alternative solution is to subcontract this out to commercial providers who therefore host your website for a fee.

For those teachers working at an established academic institution, it is worth first investigating what existing arrangements are already in place and to utilise/leverage the infrastructure that is available.

For those working at smaller institutions or looking at creating a program de novo, there are many hundreds of online commercial hosting solutions at a variety of price points. Due to the commercial and ever-changing nature of these, they are not explored in detail in this text, but further information can easily be located online if one conducts a search for 'web hosting services'.

2.7.2 Understanding 'User Interfaces' and 'Learning Management Systems'

When a learner (a human) wants to access an online learning program (digital data stored on a server), it must be presented to them in a way that they can understand and interact with. This is done via a 'user interface' (UI). The information that a learner sees on a computer screen or smartphone is the UI.

Most modern UIs are made to be extremely user-friendly. That is, the information is presented in simple, easy-to-understand ways that are intuitive to learn. However, this was not always true. Some older learners may remember early computer UIs such as MS-DOS or early mobile phones where navigating and performing tasks was onerous and text-heavy. Even in the modern era, you may be able to think of some computer programs which are more confusing and difficult to navigate than others. This is the difference between a 'good' and a 'bad' UI, and one can easily extrapolate how such differences would impact the quality of learning experiences for an online learner.

In the early days of online education, there were limited templates and commercial solutions for educational UIs and therefore educators looking to create an online learning program were often required to design their own interface.

With the rapid growth in demand for online education, it quickly became clear that there was an appetite for pre-designed UIs that were specifically created to deliver educational curricula, thereby freeing up educators to focus on the content of the programs rather than starting from scratch every time they wanted to create an online program. Hence, 'off-the-shelf' commercial educational apps and UIs have become extremely popular. These are known as 'Learning Management System (LMS).' LMSs are now so ubiquitous that bespoke learning UIs are exceptionally rare.

All major LMS solutions can now deliver a wide range of multimedia learning experiences, have interactive functionality, methods for student interaction, and methods for performing core educational administrative tasks (e.g., individual student progress-tracking, assessment uploading and scoring, time-based release of educational materials). Again, due to the rapidly evolving nature of LMSs, a deep exploration of these is not included in this manual but should be chosen based on a balance between desired functionality, user simplicity, stability, security, and cost.

2.7.3 Administrative and Support Roles

In addition to the academic team, there are numerous important administrative (Fig. 2.10) and support (Fig. 2.11) roles that are required to successfully deliver an online curriculum. Although academic staff can hold some of these roles, in the online world the increasing complexity and time required to perform these tasks means that it is often more appropriate to have separate individuals (or teams) that cover these roles.

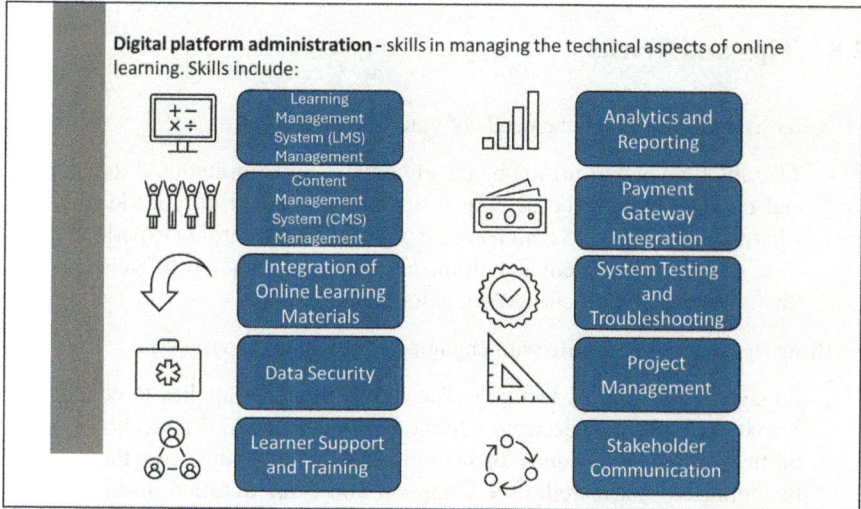

Fig. 2.10 Digital platform administration skills required in online education

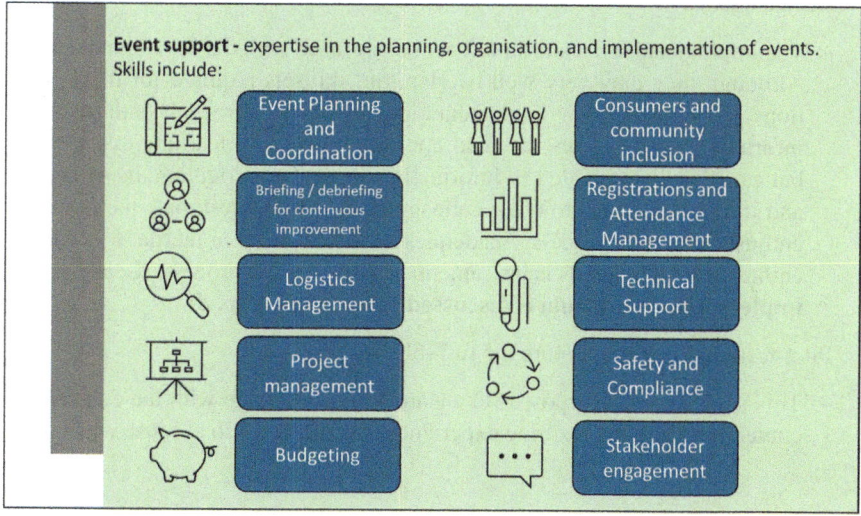

Fig. 2.11 Event support skills required in online education

Depending on how your program is structured, you may wish to have individuals who are trained and responsible for these roles internally within your program delivery team. They are also roles that can be outsourced, sometimes to professionals associated with the LMS that you have chosen. This may be the simplest option in smaller-scale programs with small staffing teams.

Like all effective teams, ensuring there is good collaboration and clear communication between team members who are involved in the different roles is vital, so that learners can be presented with a seamless experience rather than a piecemeal one.

2.8 Tips and Tricks

- Never assume you know the needs of your learners.
  - Take the time and effort to objectively obtain this information through a formal data-gathering process. The insights you glean from your learners are what will enable you to craft learning objectives and learning experiences that cater specifically to them and ultimately will make a major difference in how 'fit-for-purpose' your curriculum is for learners.
- Bring the curriculum to life with engaging educational experiences.
  - Engagement enhances learning. This simple concept applies to educational activities across the spectrum. Online education provides a wealth of possibilities for delivering education in innovative and engaging ways; these should be embraced, not feared. **(See Chaps. 4 and 5 for detailed discussions on how to do this)**.
- When assembling an implementation team, ensure a critical mass of motivated change agents.
  - The implementation team should not be confused with the development team. Although they may very well overlap, the skillsets required for these functions are separate. For implementation, you need invested, enthused, and informed change agents who can not only deliver the learning experiences, but can also disseminate key information about the curriculum, its pedagogy, and the reasons for it to other colleagues. Don't underestimate the power of enthusiasm in this process. Academics are often guilty of inertia, so a core of enthusiastic individuals is instrumental in driving this process. **(Leading and implementing curricula is discussed further in Chap. 8)**.
- Pilot-test your material before the full roll-out.
  - This serves a dual purpose – to ensure learners engage with the educational content and find the learning experiences useful, but also because when deal-

ing with any form of technology there is always the risk of IT bugs/errors with a new product. There is nothing more infuriating for a learner than sitting down to a learning experience to find that due to some unforeseen error, one cannot actually use it.

- Establish your evaluation plan upfront.
  – Evaluation runs the risk of being a 'lip-service' aspect of a curriculum, included out of necessity and with limited authentic ability to feedback into iterative curriculum design for future rollouts. This can be avoided through upfront establishment of the evaluation plan at the curriculum design stage, including a clear process for how information will 'close the curricular design loop', including how feedback is dealt with, what are the thresholds for actioning change and who is responsible for such changes.

2.9 Conclusion

Online HPE curricula design conforms to long-standing core principles of HPE curriculum design, although the implementation stage (which includes team assembly, design, and delivery of the curriculum) is a lengthier and more involved process. Utilising a systematic approach that takes into account the core theories and strategies of online education, one may develop a coherent, fit-for-purpose and effective curriculum for modern health professional learners.

References

1. Burton JL, McDonald S. Curriculum or syllabus: which are we reforming? Med Teach. 2001;23(2):187–91.
2. Kulasegaram K, Kulasegaram K, Mylopoulos M, Tonin P, Bernstein S, Bryden P, et al. The alignment imperative in curriculum renewal. Med Teach. 2018;40(5):443–8.
3. Law M, Veinot P, Mylopoulos M, Bryden P, Brydges R. Applying activity theory to undergraduate medical curriculum reform: lessons in contradictions from multiple stakeholders' perspectives. Med Teach. 2022:1–12.
4. Asch DA, Weinstein DF. Innovation in medical education. N Engl J Med. 2014;371(9):794–5.
5. Akdemir N, Malik R, Walters T, Hamstra S, Scheele F. Clinicians' perspectives on quality: do they match accreditation standards? Hum Resour Health. 2021;19(1):75.
6. World Federation for Medical Education. Basic Medical Education WFME Global Standards for Quality Improvement [Internet]. 2020 [cited 2024 Sep 18]. Available from: https://wfme.org/wp-content/uploads/2020/12/WFME-BME-Standards-2020.pdf
7. Australian Medical Council (AMC). Standards for assessment and accreditation of primary medical programs [Internet]. 2023 [cited 2024 May 12]. Available from: https://www.amc.au/wp-content/uploads/2023/08/AMC-Medical_School_Standards-FINAL.pdf
8. Roff S, McAleer S, Harden RM, Al-Qahtani M, Ahmed AU, Deza H, et al. Development and validation of the Dundee ready education environment measure (DREEM). Med Teach. 1997;19(4):295–9.

9. Norman GR. The birth and death of curricula. Adv Health Sci Educ. 2017;22(4):797–801.
10. Bordage G, Meguerditchian AN, Meguerditchian AN, Tamblyn R. Practice indicators of suboptimal care and avoidable adverse events: a content analysis of a national qualifying examination. Acad Med. 2013;88(10):1493–8.
11. Curran V, Matthews L, Fleet L, Simmons K, Gustafson DL, Wetsch LR. A review of digital, social, and mobile technologies in health professional education. J Contin Educ Health Prof. 2017;37(3):195–206.
12. Nor Azizah Binti Junida, T. Tuan, Seri Idris Jusoh. Understanding and readiness in dealing with the education transformation of the 4th industrial revolution. 2019
13. Majid FA, Ainul Azmin M, Zamin. The 4th industrial revolution: contemplations on curriculum review and its implementation in the Malaysian higher education institutes. Global J Al-Thaqafah. 2019;
14. Compton S, Sarraf-Yazdi S, Rustandy F, Radha Krishna LK. Medical students' preference for returning to the clinical setting during the COVID-19 pandemic. Med Educ. 2020;54(10):943–50.
15. Lai-Kwon J, Woodward-Kron R, Seignior D, Allen LM, McArthur G, Barrett M, et al. Qualitative evaluation of a multidisciplinary master of cancer sciences: impacts on graduates and influencing curricular factors. BMC Med Educ. 2024;
16. Koehler M, Mishra P. What is technological pedagogical content knowledge (TPACK)? Contemp Issues Technol Teacher Educ. 2009;9(1):60–70.
17. Mishra P, Koehler MJ. Technological pedagogical content knowledge: a framework for teacher knowledge. Teach Coll Rec. 2006;108(6):1017–54.
18. Hess AN. Modular online learning design: A flexible approach for diverse learning needs. American Library Association; 2020. 143 p
19. Parker AS, Steffes BC, Hill K, Bachheta N, Mangaoang D, Mwachiro M, et al. An online, modular curriculum enhances surgical education and improves learning outcomes in east, central, and southern Africa: a mixed-methods study. Ann Surg Open. 2022;3(1):e140.
20. Grunfeld E, Zitzelsberger L, Coristine M, Whelan TJ, Aspelund F, Evans WK. Job stress and job satisfaction of cancer care workers. Psycho-Oncol. 2005;14(1):61–9.
21. Hollis RB, Was CA. Mind wandering, control failures, and social media distractions in online learning. Learn Instr. 2016;42:104–12.
22. Guo PJ, Kim J, Rubin R. How video production affects student engagement: an empirical study of MOOC videos. In: Proceedings of the first ACM conference on Learning @ scale conference; Atlanta, GA, USA; 2014.
23. Peters GW, Ford E, Burmeister J, Juang T, Lincoln H, Brown D, et al. Lessons learned from multi-institutional medical physics animated video production. University of Chicago; 2022. p. 24.
24. Rose DH, Harbour WS, Johnston CS, Daley SG, Abarbanell L. Universal design for learning in postsecondary education: reflections on principles and their application. J Postsecond Educ Dis. 2006;19(2):135–51.
25. Kok DL, Dushyanthen S, Giuliani M, Garda AE, Golden DW. Chapter 106—education to translate research into practice. In: Eltorai AEM, Bakal JA, Kim DW, Wazer DE, editors. Translational radiation oncology [Internet]. Academic Press; 2023. p. 647–52. Cited 2024 May 25 (Handbook for Designing and Conducting Clinical and Translational Research). Available from: https://www.sciencedirect.com/science/article/pii/B9780323884235001047.
26. Stufflebeam DL, McCormick CH, Brinkerhoff RO, Nelson CO. Conducting educational needs assessments, vol. 10. Springer Science & Business Media; 2012.
27. McCawley PF. Methods for conducting an educational needs assessment. University of Idaho. 2009;23(6–14)
28. Chatterjee D, Corral J. How to write well-defined learning objectives. J Educ Perioper Med. 2017;19(4)

29. Lai-Kwon J, Dushyanthen S, Seignior D, Barrett M, Buisman-Pijlman F, Buntine A, et al. Designing a wholly online, multidisciplinary master of cancer sciences degree. BMC Med Educ. 2023;23(1):544.
30. Popenici S, Millar V. Writing learning outcomes: a practical guide for academics. Melbourne Centre for the Study of Higher Education, The University of Melbourne; 2015
31. Harden RM, Davis MH. AMEE Medical Education Guide No. 5. The core curriculum with options or special study modules. Med Teach. 1995;17(2):125–48.
32. Biggs J. Enhancing teaching through constructive alignment. High Educ. 1996;32(3):347–64.
33. Crossley JGM. Addressing learner disorientation: give them a roadmap. Med Teach. 2014;36(8):685–91.
34. Akdemir N, Ellwood D, Walters T, Scheele F. Accreditation as a quality improvement tool: is it still relevant? Med J Aust. 2018;209(6):249–52.
35. Hedrick JS, Cottrell S, Stark D, Brownfield E, Stoddard HA, Angle SM, et al. A review of continuous quality improvement processes at ten medical schools. Med Sci Educator. 2019;29(1):285–90.
36. Morrison J. Evaluation. BMJ. 2003;326(7385):385–7.
37. Schiekirka S, Feufel MA, Herrmann-Lingen C, Raupach T. Evaluation in medical education: a topical review of target parameters, data collection tools and confounding factors. Ger Med Sci. 2015;
38. Boyle P, Grimm M, Scicluna H, McNeil HP. The UNSW medicine student experience questionnaire (MedSEQ): a synopsis of its development, features and utility. 2009;
39. Huang PH, Velan G, Smith G, Fentoullis M, Kennedy SE, Gibson KJ, et al. What impacts students' satisfaction the most from medicine student experience questionnaire in Australia: a validity study. J Educ Eval Health Prof. 2023;20:2.
40. Velthuis F, Varpio L, Helmich E, Dekker H, Jaarsma ADC. Navigating the complexities of undergraduate medical curriculum change: change leaders' perspectives. Acad Med. 2018;93(10):1503.
41. Ezzati M, Martin H, Skjold S, Vander Hoorn S, Murray CJL. Trends in national and state-level obesity in the USA after correction for self-report bias: analysis of health surveys. J R Soc Med. 2006;99(5):250–7.
42. Allen LM, Hay M, Palermo C. Evaluation in health professions education-is measuring outcomes enough? Med Educ. 2021;
43. Pock AR, Williams PM, Maranich AM, Landoll RR, Witkop CT, Reamy BV, et al. Curricular change and resiliency in the era of coronavirus (COVID-19): the Uniformed Services University of the Health Sciences (USU) experience. Mil Med. 2021;186(1–2):212–8.
44. Kraakevik JA, Frederick M, Ryan N, Haedinger LA, Carney PA. An observational study of an approach to accommodate a fourth-year to third-year neurology clerkship curricular transition. Med Educ Online. 2020;25(1):1710331.
45. White J, Paslawski T, Kearney RA. "Discovery Learning": an account of rapid curriculum change in response to accreditation. Med Teach. 2013;35(7)
46. Arja SB, Arja SB, Venkata MR, Nayakanti A, Kottathveetil P, Acharya Y. Integrated curriculum and the change process in undergraduate medical education. Med Teach. 2018;40(5):437–42.
47. Katajavuori N, Salminen O, Vuorensola K, Huhtala H, Vuorela P, Hirvonen J. Competence-based pharmacy education in the University of Helsinki. Pharmacy. 2017;5(2):29.
48. Aagaard E, Yau T, Dufault C. Curriculum renewal in the time of COVID-19: the Washington University School of Medicine Story. FASEB bioAdv. 2020;3(3):143–9.
49. Kok DL, Dushyanthen S, Peters G, Sapkaroski D, Barrett M, Sim J, et al. Screen-based digital learning methods in radiation oncology education—a review and expert commentary. Technical innovations and patient support. Radiat Oncol. 2022;

Chapter 3
Contexts and Conditions for Online Learning Success

Michelle Barrett, David Seignior, and Alicia Mew

Abstract Online learning offers opportunities to enhance health professional education (HPE), by facilitating collaborative knowledge sharing, communication, and peer networking in education, training, and continuing professional development and support. But online learning does not just happen online, it takes place in both virtual and physical spaces, including the clinical workplace, all of which influence the nature of the learning experience. It is important to understand the wider context in which online learning is situated and factors such as technology, organisational culture, and learner demographics and motivations, need to be considered when designing and delivering accessible and inclusive HPE online education.

Key Points Online Learning

- Supports collaborative knowledge sharing, communication, and networking, essential for health professional education (HPE), training and development.
- Is shaped by and includes technology, social interactions, organisational cultures, demographics, societal norms, individual motivations and both physical and virtual spaces.
- Requires intentional instructional design that establishes clear goals, strategic alignment, adaptive learning technologies, and contextualised activities.
- Leverages synchronous (live, real-time interaction) and asynchronous (self-paced, recorded) modalities across in-person, online, blended, and multimodal formats.
- Enhances workplace learning through convenience, personalisation, interactivity, and collaboration.
- Depends on community-building tools like collaborative projects, discussion forums, and social learning networks to promote motivation and active learning.

M. Barrett (✉) · A. Mew
Victorian Comprehensive Cancer Centre, Melbourne, VIC, Australia
e-mail: michelle.barrett@unimelb.edu.au

D. Seignior
University of Melbourne, Melbourne, VIC, Australia

- Must support diverse learner backgrounds through cultural and linguistic inclusivity, accessibility features, online support, and equitable resources.

3.1 Introduction

Online learning refers to a learning environment facilitated by internet-based technology. However, although it sounds counterintuitive, online learning is never just online; it occurs in both virtual and physical spaces, including workplaces and homes. It is crucial to consider the interplay between online learning contexts and in-person experiences, whether in educational or workplace settings. This chapter will discuss asynchronous and synchronous forms of engagement, wholly online and blended learning formats, and their application in training, education, continuing professional development, and support. Emphasis will be on the role of a learning culture (social presence), intentional content (cognitive presence), and a professional educator (teacher presence) to ensure effective online learning.

The scope of online learning contexts in health professional education is extensive and includes various modalities and formats. Chapter 4 delves deeper into technology-enhanced instructional practices.

The benefits of online learning depend on a range of broader contexts: institutional, societal, cultural, technological, personal, psychological, physical, economic, political, and global. These contexts and their benefits are seen from the perspectives of learners, educators, institutions, and society. HPE can use technology to enhance communication and knowledge exchange, allowing for collaboration, networking, and the dissemination of up-to-date medical science and clinical practice. This allows learners to actively participate in constructing their own knowledge and engaging with diverse perspectives, leading to a deeper, well-rounded understanding of medical concepts and real-world applications.

This chapter provides an overview of online learning contexts in HPE, exploring their definition, scope, roles, benefits, barriers, enablers, practical considerations, and future applications. In subsequent chapters, we will delve into the methods, tools, and techniques that underpin technology-enhanced instructional practices. By integrating an array of modalities and formats into HPE curricula, we can harness the transformative potential of technology-enabled networks in fostering communication, collaboration, rapid content consolidation, and knowledge exchange among health professionals.

3.2 Understanding the Online Context

Learning happens when our brains store new information from our experiences or thoughts [1]. The context, or the setting and circumstances in which something occurs, plays a crucial role in this process [2]. When we talk about a learning context, we are referring to the specific environment or situation that makes acquiring knowledge meaningful and applicable. Originating from the Latin word 'contexere' the term 'context' means "to weave together" [3].

Before formal schooling and vocational training were commonplace, people learned through their daily interactions and activities. This approach to learning is still seen today in apprenticeships, cadetships, and other types of on-the-job training. However, during the era of Taylorism (a systematic approach to improving industrial efficiency), education became more standardised, with a focus on delivering uniform content from teacher to student, neglecting the importance of individualised, contextual learning [4]. This method assumed that knowing and doing were separate, a position now countered by the understanding that knowledge is deeply connected to the specific activities and contexts in which it is used [5–7].

In today's digital age, an online learning context means using technology to facilitate education. This includes not just the digital tools and platforms, but also the social interactions, organisational culture, and various physical and virtual spaces that influence how learners experience and perceive their education [8, 9]. Understanding this online context is vital because it affects how well learners can acquire, retain, and use new knowledge and skills. By recognising these factors, educators can curate an optimal learning environment to enhance educational outcomes [10].

3.3 Role in the Global Workplace

The rapid rise of online technologies has provided educators with a platform to standardise and democratise education across geographic, racial, cultural, societal, and economic borders [11, 12]. UNESCO (United Nations Educational, Scientific and Cultural Organisation with the mission to promote international collaborations in education, science, culture, and communication), has acknowledged online learning's role in the formation of a stable society by including it within the sustainable development goals [13].

In dynamic environments like healthcare, the amalgamation of online learning with traditional workplace learning has emerged as an efficient and transformational learning modality for adapting to this agile setting, particularly for healthcare professionals with multifaceted roles and diverse learning needs [14]. Online learning enhances workplace learning by offering advantages such as convenience, personalisation, interactivity, and collaboration [15, 16]. Adult learners, commonly engaging in both online and workplace learning simultaneously, require tailored strategies to attain proficiency in their roles [17]. Unlike formal learning environments, workplace learning often unfolds informally, relying heavily on social interactions and individual development [6, 18].

Effective workplace learning happens when learners have control, access to resources, and are actively engaged with their work [19]. Healthcare professional's individual attributes and the contextual factors within their work environment, such as social relationships, power dynamics, and expectations, exert significant influence on learning outcomes [20]. Peer reflection is critical to the learning process [21], and online platforms facilitate such collaborative endeavours through collaboration and knowledge sharing [15, 22].

3.4 Building Blocks and Best Practices: Navigating the Online Learning Landscape

When designing and implementing online learning within the healthcare sector, success relies on understanding and navigating its various critical components. These include: the instructional design of the learning experience, dynamics of social interactions, nuances of organisational culture and structures, demographic considerations, personal motivators and drivers, societal constructs, and the interplay between physical and virtual spaces (**see** Fig. 3.1). Understanding these building blocks and embracing best practices is essential for healthcare professionals navigating the online learning landscape.

3.4.1 Instructional Design of the Learning Experience

When implementing instructional design in HPE, educators often think only of designing a curriculum to impart discipline-specific knowledge and skills (**as discussed in detail in** Chap. 2). However, beyond these factors, there are principles and values conveyed to the learner implicitly through instructional design decisions. These may, in turn, influence learners' perceptions of the relevance and desirability of the learning experience, as well as whether they apply the learnings.

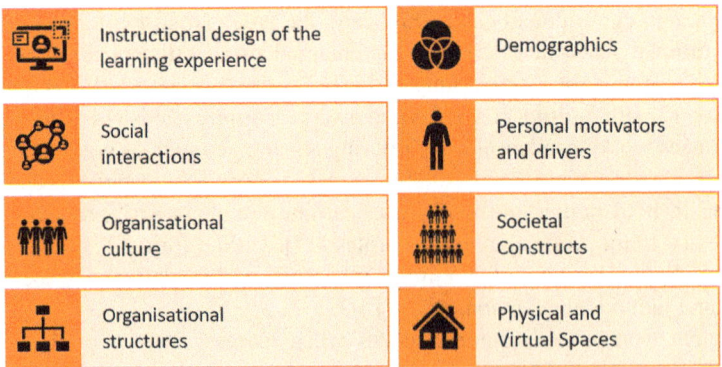

Fig. 3.1 The contextual 'building blocks' that influence online learning

	Resource Allocation	Provide financial, human and time resources to educators and their teams to enhance their teaching effectiveness.
	Strategic alignment and standardisation	Connect universities, healthcare, and research organisations through partnerships, academic roles, and standard systems helps create consistent and scalable teaching methods.
	Curriculum and content development	Create a curriculum with clear learning objectives aligned to course design, constructive alignment and evidence-based content ensures engaging and relevant learning experiences.
	Adaptive learning and accessibility	Use adaptive learning technologies and feedback mechanisms provides tailored educational experiences for all learners.
	Community building & collaborative practice	Foster a collaborative community of practice among educators and learners encourages shared knowledge and peer support.
	Contextualisation and empowerment	Design learning activities that empower learners and integrate practical, real-world contexts enhances knowledge transfer into practice.

Fig. 3.2 Supportive practices for aligning instructional design with online learning

For instance, learning designs that are inclusive, accessible, and collaborative increase the potential audience of an online degree (which is, by nature, not limited by geographic boundaries). Curricular choices can (and should), therefore, reflect organisational values, for instance, including diverse educators, flexible learning arrangements, involving consumers, or prioritising learning methods that promote eco-friendliness [23].

Supportive practices for aligning instructional design with online learning are described in Fig. 3.2.

Instructional design of effective online learning experiences requires appropriate resources, structures, constructive alignment, and design elements to connect and contextualise the content within the health professional's work environment.

3.4.2 Social Interactions

Social interactions between learners, educators, and peers help shape the learning experience. Engaging in discussions, sharing perspectives, providing feedback, and peer assessment can all contribute to a strong sense of agency, community enjoyment, connection, and support amongst learners and educators.

Supportive practices for aligning social interactions with online learning are described in Fig. 3.3.

Effective facilitation of social interactions is essential to promote active learning, engagement and adherence, peer teaching, and the exchange of diverse ideas and viewpoints.

💬	Engagement & ice-breaking	Integrate icebreakers and introductions to build rapport.
💻	Communication & interaction tools	Utilise real-life chat platforms, polling, word clouds, question and answer opportunities, synchronous webinars, tutorials and directed instruction with breakout rooms for dynamic participation.
👥	Collaborative learning	Integrate collaborative group projects with real-world relevance, discussion forums, co-authoring, learner presentations, peer review, brainstorming tools and appointment of trained educators to facilitate collaborative learning.
🔗	Social learning networks	Create course-specific social groups, community of practices and integration of social media platforms for a more connected learning experience.
⭐	Recognition & motivation strategies	Communicate learner achievements and implementing badging, reward and recognition schemes for motivation.

Fig. 3.3 Supportive practices for aligning social interactions with online learning

3.4.3 Organisational Culture

The organisational culture of a healthcare, research, or educational institution significantly shapes the online learning environment [8], and impacts service performance, quality, safety, and improvement [24]. Organisational culture reflects values, beliefs, and commitment to education through investment in resources, technology, and its people. If online learning is reflected in organisational policies and practices, strategic planning, and vision and mission statements, there will be a higher probability that the latest technologies, pedagogical approaches, and priority for workplace learning will be adopted [25].

Supportive practices for aligning organisational culture with online learning are described in Fig. 3.4.

Organisational culture influences the success of online learning integration in healthcare. By fostering a culture that values innovative and learner-centred approaches, organisations demonstrate their commitment to employee development. This then translates into higher staff satisfaction, retention, and advancement opportunities. By supporting the integration of online learning, organisations invest in their workforce's growth, driving continuous improvement in healthcare delivery and ultimately improving patient outcomes.

3.4.4 Organisational Structures

The organisational structure of an institution significantly influences the implementation and sustainability of online learning initiatives [26]. Effective leadership at all levels is crucial in providing a clear vision, strategic direction, and culture of innovation and educational excellence [27]. Advocating for appropriate budgetary

	Culture of growth	Emphasise online learning in vision, mission statements emphasising assessment, feedback and quality assurance, to reflect an organisational growth and renewal culture.
	Professional development	Provide opportunities for skill and knowledge expansion through training, educational programs and research projects.
	Resource allocation	Address economic barriers with sponsorships, scholarships and significant resources for integrating online tools and methodologies.
	Organisational infrastructure & alignment	Establish specialised departments, learning and content management systems for internal and external access, to foster a culture that embraces and advances online learning.
	Academic support	Offer university affiliations, academic appointments and research support to enhance academic stature of individuals and the organisation.
	Quality assurance & recognition	Maintain high educational standards and celebrate achievements through recognition programs.
	Community building & inclusivity	Foster a supportive educational network with inclusive practice for diverse learners.
	Global engagement and cultural exchange	Provide international placements and cultural exchange programs for personal and professional development.

Fig. 3.4 Supportive practices for aligning organisational culture with online learning

allocation enables the acquisition of technology, develops and maintains content, provides educational opportunities, trains educators, and ensures infrastructure and support systems are embedded and effective [28]. Human resource policies and established networks can also support the recruitment and retention of skilled online learning professionals.

Supportive practices for aligning organisational structures with online learning are described in Fig. 3.5.

An organisation that is well-structured, with leadership alignment, opportunities for departmental connectivity, adequate budgetary and human resource allocation, credible reward and recognition programs, robust strategic partnerships, and a commitment to quality, is poised for success in establishing an effective and enduring online learning environment.

3.4.5 Demographics

The readiness and motivation of learners to engage with online learning significantly influences whether the initiative will be successful or not [29]. Often additional support is needed to bridge divides for specific demographics, or individual learner, needs.

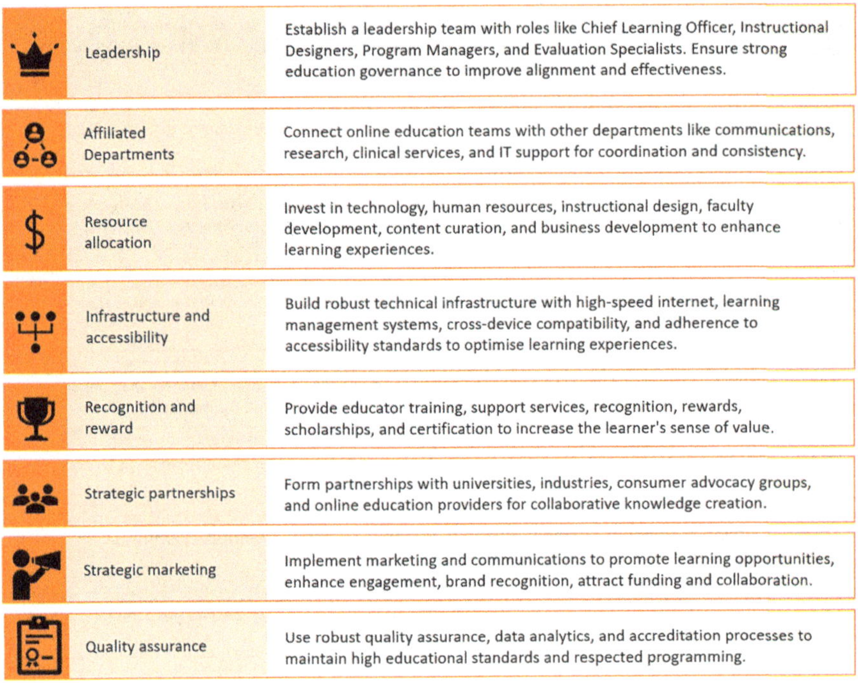

♛	Leadership	Establish a leadership team with roles like Chief Learning Officer, Instructional Designers, Program Managers, and Evaluation Specialists. Ensure strong education governance to improve alignment and effectiveness.
👥	Affiliated Departments	Connect online education teams with other departments like communications, research, clinical services, and IT support for coordination and consistency.
$	Resource allocation	Invest in technology, human resources, instructional design, faculty development, content curation, and business development to enhance learning experiences.
	Infrastructure and accessibility	Build robust technical infrastructure with high-speed internet, learning management systems, cross-device compatibility, and adherence to accessibility standards to optimise learning experiences.
🏆	Recognition and reward	Provide educator training, support services, recognition, rewards, scholarships, and certification to increase the learner's sense of value.
👥	Strategic partnerships	Form partnerships with universities, industries, consumer advocacy groups, and online education providers for collaborative knowledge creation.
📢	Strategic marketing	Implement marketing and communications to promote learning opportunities, enhance engagement, brand recognition, attract funding and collaboration.
📋	Quality assurance	Use robust quality assurance, data analytics, and accreditation processes to maintain high educational standards and respected programming.

Fig. 3.5 Supportive practices for aligning organisational structures with online learning

Learner demographics to be considered include gender, educational background, cultural heritage, language proficiency, health specialisation, job role, geographical location, (dis)ability and experiences. Understanding the diverse demographics of learners is crucial for designing inclusive and equitable online learning experiences. It requires tailoring content and instruction to meet the unique needs and preferences of the individual learners to enhance engagement, accessibility, a sense of belonging, and cross-cultural understanding. The demographics of the educators can also heavily influence the learning experience (43).

Supportive practices for aligning learner demographics with online learning are described in Fig. 3.6.

Inclusivity and accessibility are key considerations in acknowledging and addressing the diverse cultural, linguistic, and educational needs of learners and educators in the online context.

💬	Cultural and linguistic inclusion	Offer cultural competency training, multilingual resources, inclusive curriculum design, cultural perspective sharing, flexible scheduling, customisable learning pathways, and feedback integration.
🧑‍🏫	Representative educational leadership	Recruit leaders and educators who reflect or challenge learner demographics to foster an inclusive curriculum and teaching approach.
♿	Accessibility and support	Provide accessibility training for educators, 24/7 culturally competent tech support, English as a second language (ESL) support, development of online and information literacy skills, and flexible assessment strategies.
🔗	Equitable Access and Resources	Ensure technology access through scholarships, loan devices, subsidies, and mentorship programs to support diverse learners.

Fig. 3.6 Supportive practices for aligning learner demographics with online learning

3.4.6 Personal Motivators and Drivers

Health professional engagement with online learning contexts is influenced by unique motivators and drivers specific to their personality type, skill sets, occupational roles, and setting. Bandura's Social Cognitive Theory (SCT), states that to achieve desired results, a learner must have high levels of self-efficacy, or belief in their own ability to organise and act [30] and that this perception is based on their evaluation of their previous outcomes [31]. The role of self-efficacy in predicting positive online learning outcomes has been proven in adult learners [8]. A healthcare professional's confidence and skill in using a computer and the internet greatly affects their effective utilisation and engagement with online learning [32].

Online learning enables health professionals to keep abreast of rapidly evolving information driven by new research, technology, and treatment modalities. In turn, health professionals can practice risk-free procedures and patient care without fear of patient harm or reprisal. Access is available just in time and at all hours to accommodate busy schedules and needs. Platforms enable connection with colleagues to learn from each other across cultural and geographical divides, fostering collaboration and allowing for global dissemination of information and influence. Integration of effective online learning in training programs leads to enhanced engagement with online platforms in the workplace, such as electronic medical records, telehealth platforms, machine learning-assisted diagnostics, gene editing technologies, etc.

Supportive practices for aligning learner motivators and drivers with online learning are described in Fig. 3.7.

Although extremely important, access to a well-designed and well-resourced online learning environment is not sufficient to ensure learner engagement. The learner's approach, reflection, consolidation, and connection of the content to their work are imperative for achieving learning outcomes and ensuring it is incorporated into practice.

	Contextualisation and relevance	Ensure learning objectives are embedded in real-world scenarios through robust content curation and strategic partnerships.
	High quality resources and accessibility	Provide access to high-quality, relevant resources by supporting both formal and informal learning and co-producing materials with strategic partners.
	Knowledge translation	Enhance knowledge translation into applied skills through interactive elements like discussion forums, webinars, and gamification.
	Networking	Support community-based learning outcomes by creating communities of practice and integrating collaborative tools.
	Strategic partnerships	Foster co-designed knowledge creation and scholarship through affiliations and partnerships with universities and industry groups.
	Recognition and incentivisation	Promote learner motivation and highlight achievements through accreditation, badging, and reward schemes.

Fig. 3.7 Supportive practices for aligning learner motivators and drivers with online learning

3.4.7 Societal Constructs

The successful integration and uptake of online learning are deeply influenced by various societal constructs such as ethics, laws, politics, and the economy. Ethical considerations, including privacy, data security, and academic integrity, play a crucial role in ensuring a trustworthy online learning environment. Legal regulations impact everything from content accessibility and intellectual property rights to commercialisation, professional behaviours, and accreditation standards. Political decisions at organisational, state, and federal levels can significantly shape the implementation, access, and funding of online learning programs. Additionally, economic factors determine the affordability and availability of online learning opportunities, financial aid options, and the cost of necessary technology. Together, these societal constructs create a complex interplay that influence how effectively online learning can be accessed, adopted, and utilised.

Supportive practices for aligning societal constructs with online learning are described in Fig. 3.8.

Awareness of societal constructs is crucial in ensuring that online learning experiences are ethically sound, compliant with relevant laws, politically savvy, and economically feasible. Striking a balance between educational objectives and these constructs is essential for the responsible and effective implementation of online learning.

⚖️	Regulatory compliance and ethics	Ensure an ethical and compliant learning environment through online learning policies, academic integrity training, legal awareness, respectful behaviour promotion, and privacy or security protocols.
👨‍🏫	Accessibility and inclusivity	Guarantee inclusive and accessible online learning with open access, single sign-on registration, financial support, cost transparency, data privacy, literacy training, and outreach to underserved communities.
$	Financial considerations	Support financial viability of online learning by creating commercialisation opportunities, conducting economic analyses, and incorporating partnerships, mentorship, traineeships, and employment initiatives.
⁂	Strategic relationships and advocacy	Ensure integration, growth, and sustainability through global collaborations, corporate partnerships, and political advocacy for online learning.

Fig. 3.8 Supportive practices for aligning societal constructs with online learning

3.4.8 Physical and Virtual Spaces

The physical and virtual spaces surrounding learners and educators in an online learning context significantly influence their experiences and perceptions [9, 18]. The physical environment includes the location where learners engage with online content, such as an office, laboratory, classroom, library, home setting, or whilst in transit. The technical space includes the hardware, software, and internet connectivity that learners and educators use to access online resources. The hardware includes the tools and devices available, such as computers, tablets, headsets, virtual reality headsets, and mobile devices. The interplay of these spaces can influence learner and educator accessibility, comfort, and convenience, which in turn affects the learning experience and outcomes.

Supportive practices for aligning physical and virtual spaces with online learning are described in Fig. 3.9.

Integrating online learning into organisation and education settings requires consideration from the perspectives of learners, educators, supervisors, educational institutions, workplaces, and society. By addressing these dimensions, learners can engage effectively with online learning materials and activities, promoting a positive and productive educational experience.

3.5 Modalities and Formats

The different types of modalities and formats utilised within health professional education are expansive, encompassing a wide range of applications and tools. It includes online courses and modules that cover fundamental medical knowledge, specialised clinical skills, and up-to-date healthcare practices.

The three different types of learning modalities utilised over the past few decades have included (1) in-person, where traditionally the educator and learner are

	Infrastructure and accessibility	Establish robust technical infrastructure that includes high-speed internet, servers, user-friendly learning systems, and flexible, accessible designs to optimise learning experiences.
	Support and usability	Provide 24/7 technical support, clear guidance on hardware/software, online library access, and ensure privacy and data protection for a secure learning environment.
	Interactive and engaging content	Incorporate engaging materials, virtual labs, simulations, and social learning activities to make online learning immersive.
	Community and collaboration	Promote remote supervision, online communities of practice, collaborative tools, and virtual campus experiences to foster a sense of community.
	Continuous improvement and training	Regularly update systems, act on feedback, and provide online literacy training to continuously enhance online learning for both learners and educators.

Fig. 3.9 Supportive practices for aligning physical and virtual spaces with online learning

co-located; (2) blended or hybrid which combines in-person and online; and (3) online, where all learning is enabled by technology and occurs remotely [33].

Online learning leverages synchronous (live, real-time interaction) and asynchronous (self-paced, recorded) modalities across in-person, online, blended, and multimodal formats. Historically tied to in-person delivery, synchronous learning now includes live-streaming and online tutorials [8], whereas asynchronous learning uses online systems for flexible, self-paced access to content.

Formats can include social media platforms, microlearning, online courses, continuing medical education, symposia, conferences, webinars, podcasts, workshops, online learning modules and courses, micro-credentialled courses, massive open online courses (MOOCs), internships, fellowships, traineeships, virtual simulations, mentorship programs, applications, blogs, interactive resources, and higher degree award courses.

3.6 Patient Centredness

To ensure healthcare education is patient-centred in its approach, educators must consider innovative ways of integrating the patient and their support networks (consumers), into online learning design, implementation, evaluation, and recognition [34]. For example, Australia has a strong commitment to a healthcare system based on partnerships with consumers [34]. Strategies include consumers as educators, co-designers, reviewers, facilitators, presenters, assessors, simulated patients, panellists, interviewers, selectors, discussion board commentators, storytellers, faculty members, education researchers, coaches, curriculum collaborators, and as fellow participants learning alongside health professionals and sharing the wisdom of their perspectives. Gathering consumer perspectives can also be elicited through surveys, focus groups, consumer networks, interviews, and reflective journals. It is imperative that there is educator and consumer training, consumer support systems, consumer representation at all levels of governance, consumer remuneration, and consumer networks or communities of practice, to create a sense of value and empowerment for the consumer, their collaborating education colleagues, and the learners.

3.6.1 An Applied Example of Embedding the Patient as Person Module

The "Patient as a Person" (PAP) Module is an example of how involving consumers can enhance educational programming for healthcare professionals. This innovative program brought together consumer educators and undergraduate students from nine different health professional fields, spanning three educational institutions. The focus of the PAP Module was on the profound impact chronic conditions have on the social and mental well-being of patients and their support networks.

Groups consisting of 12 health profession students—representing disciplines such as medicine, health sciences, public health, physiotherapy, occupational therapy, nursing, speech therapy, art therapy, and homecare—joined four consumers with diverse chronic disease backgrounds. These groups met three times to share experiences and insights.

The consumers participating in the program made several insightful recommendations to improve its effectiveness, which included: (1) centralising consumer recruitment through a single entity to streamline the process across multiple organisations; (2) the importance of ensuring consumers are well-informed about the program and the learners' backgrounds to create a sense of community, gratitude, and value; (3) centralising facilitator training and aligning assessment tasks while allowing for some flexibility to match different organisational curricula, (4) empowering both student and consumer leaders, and (5) clearly defining the roles and responsibilities between the central coordinating organisation and the educational institutions involved [35].

An evaluation of the PAP Module highlighted the benefits of consumer involvement that included improved self-management, better insights into their preferences, increased peer support, improved self-acceptance, a renewed sense of purpose, and developed a more coherent and less emotional illness narrative. In terms of shared decision-making, consumers appreciated the importance of sharing their expertise about their bodies, became more assertive, and gained insights into the perspectives of healthcare professionals. This resulted in more equal relationships with healthcare providers and greater control over their healthcare trajectories [36].

To provide the necessary infrastructure and support for this program, the "Mens Achter de Patient" (MAP) or the Patient as a Person Foundation was established.

This Foundation played a crucial role in consumer recruitment, communication, and orientation. It coordinated the logistics and finances of the educational programs across participating institutions and provided training for teachers on delivering and assessing the PAP Module and similar educational initiatives.

3.7 Impact on Equity

Educational justice is the sense of honouring and valuing every student and teacher's cultural, linguistic, and historical backgrounds [37]. It espouses open-mindedness to alternative perspectives, inviting a critique of pre-established beliefs so there is a shift toward equity.

Online learning has the potential to enhance educational equity by providing access to diverse learners across different geographical, social, and economic backgrounds. It offers flexible learning options and allows traditional barriers such as distance and physical accessibility to be navigated, serving as a powerful vehicle for inclusion. It is important to ensure accessibility and inclusion for people with disabilities, such as visual impairment through adherence to Web Content Accessibility Guidelines (WCAG) (61). This accessibility is crucial in reaching underserved areas and marginalised learner communities, potentially reducing educational disparities and supporting a more diverse workforce. However, accommodating this diverse learning cohort requires careful design and implementation to ensure content is culturally relevant and accessible, irrespective of learning needs.

Online education bridges gaps whilst presenting new challenges that can exacerbate existing inequalities. Technological limitations, such as inadequate internet access and lack of digital devices, disproportionately affect those in lower socio-economic areas, widening the educational divide. Digital literacy and the need for specialised training for both learners and educators are also critical considerations that need addressing to capitalise on the benefits of online learning.

Effective online learning environments require inclusive teaching practices that value the cultural, linguistic, and historical backgrounds of every student and teacher [37]. These environments encourage open-mindedness, a re-evaluation of pre-established beliefs, and a shift to more equitable educational practices. Strategies include collaboration among educators, an adaptation of learning materials, and individualised student support to enhance the learning experience and foster an inclusive culture.

To promote educational equity through online learning, it is essential to magnify the enablers and address the barriers effectively. This requires the involvement of all stakeholders in a concerted effort to develop and implement solutions that are not only technologically sound but also culturally and linguistically tailored to meet the diverse needs of the learner population. If done according to best practices, online learning can not only increase access to education but also contribute to a more equitable and just educational landscape.

3.8 Tips and Tricks

- When designing online learning, undertake an 'audit' of the wider contexts in which it will take place, including institutional attitudes and values, leaders and advocates, and organisational strategic alignment, to optimise chances of success.
- Map out other contextual factors, such as virtual and physical learning spaces and technologies needed by both teachers and learners, then choose the relevant modality i.e., wholly online or blended.
- Integrate work-based learning into the curriculum, including case studies and practice-based learning, that allows for real world application of knowledge and skills.
- Create 'learner personas' that identify the diverse needs of your potential learners, including cultural and linguistic backgrounds, gender, (dis)ability, and socio-economic contexts.
- Ensure accessibility for all learners, including those with visual impairments. Refer to WCAG for guidelines (61).

3.9 Conclusion

The evolving landscape of online learning presents unprecedented opportunities for health professional education, fundamentally reshaping how knowledge is acquired, shared, and applied. By understanding and leveraging diverse online learning contexts, educational institutions can provide flexible, scalable, and impactful learning experiences. The integration of technology into education supports the development of essential skills and knowledge, fostering a collaborative, inclusive, and innovative environment for learners and educators alike.

Embracing the principles of the Community of Inquiry (COI) Framework—cognitive, social, and educator presence—ensures that online learning contexts are effective and meaningful. Addressing barriers and enablers, and recognising the importance of organisational culture, social interactions, and learner demographics, are essential for creating an inclusive and supportive educational ecosystem. The dynamic growth of online learning technologies promises to enhance interactivity, personalisation, and engagement, further democratising education and empowering healthcare professionals to stay at the forefront of their field.

As we navigate the future of health professional education, it is imperative to continually adapt and innovate, harnessing the full potential of online learning. By doing so, we can ensure that education remains accessible, relevant, and transformative, equipping healthcare professionals with the skills and knowledge needed to deliver high-quality care in an ever-changing world.

References

1. Speelman CP, Kirsner K. Beyond the learning curve: the construction of mind. Oxford: Oxford University Press; 2005. 288 p
2. https://www.collinsdictionary.com/dictionary/english/context#:~:text=The%20context%20 of%20a%20word,relation%20More%20Synonyms%20of%20context
3. Figueiredo AD d. Learning contexts: a blueprint for research. Interact Educ Multimed. 2005:127–39.
4. De Figueiredo AD, Afonso AP, editors. Managing learning in virtual settings: the role of context [Internet]. IGI Global; 2006. [Cited 2024 Jun 4]. Available from: http://services.igi-global. com/resolvedoi/resolve.aspx?doi=10.4018/978-1-59140-488-0
5. Billet S. Learning through work: workplace affordances and individual engagement. J Workplace Learn. 13(5):209–14.
6. Tynjälä P. Toward a 3-P model of workplace learning: a literature review. Vocat Learn. 2013 Apr;6(1):11–36.
7. Wenger E. Communities of practice: learning, meaning, and identity [Internet]. Cambridge University Press; 1999. [cited 2024 Jun 3]. Available from: https://books.google.com.au/boo ks?hl=en&lr=&id=heBZpgYUKdAC&oi=fnd&pg=PP15&dq=Wenger,E.(1999),Communiti esofPractice:Learning,Meaning,andIdentity,CambridgeUniversity+Press,Cambridge.&ots=k hlh-kgw0j&sig=2IlnykC8LgiQlPp__Ulz3GvCGXE
8. Kumar P, Kumar N, Ting H. An impact of content delivery, equity, support and self-efficacy on student's learning during the COVID-19. Curr Psychol. 2023;42(3):2460–70.
9. Alzahrani HA, Shati AA, Bawahab MA, Alamri AA, Hassan B, Patel AA, et al. Students' perception of asynchronous versus synchronous distance learning during COVID-19 pandemic in a medical college, southwestern region of Saudi Arabia. BMC Med Educ. 2023;23(1):53.
10. Roque L, Almeida A, Figueiredo AD. Context engineering: an IS development research agenda. ECIS 2004 Proc. 2004:111.
11. Mishra L, Gupta T, Shree A. Online teaching-learning in higher education during lockdown period of COVID-19 pandemic. Int J Educ Res Open. 2020;1:100012.
12. Zheng F, Khan NA, Hussain S. The COVID 19 pandemic and digital higher education: exploring the impact of proactive personality on social capital through internet self-efficacy and online interaction quality. Child Youth Serv Rev. 2020;119:105694.
13. Farah L. Entertainment and information industries. In World economic forum. Available at Accessed 5 Sept 2020. 2020
14. McCutcheon K, O'Halloran P, Lohan M. Online learning versus blended learning of clinical supervisee skills with pre-registration nursing students: a randomised controlled trial. Int J Nurs Stud. 2018;82:30–9.
15. Karakas F, Manisaligil A. Reorienting self-directed learning for the creative digital era. Eur J Train Dev. 2012;36(7):712–31.
16. Littlejohn A, Beetham H, McGill L. Learning at the digital frontier: a review of digital literacies in theory and practice. J Comput Assist Learn. 2012;28(6):547–56.
17. Cross J. Informal learning: rediscovering the natural pathways that inspire innovation and performance [Internet]. Wiley; 2011. [cited 2024 Jun 14]. Available from: https://books.google. com.au/books?hl=en&lr=&id=S38te9Z6OpoC&oi=fnd&pg=PT9&dq=Crouse,+P.,+Doyle,+ M.,+%26+Young,+M.+(2011).+Informal+learning:+Rediscovering+the+natural+pathways+t hat+inspire+innovation+and+performance.+Wiley.+&ots=EszzP0k1IN&sig=3AYdMmIbu5T dplMvOh3mI8i3YM4
18. Ng CF. The physical learning environment of online distance learners in higher education—a conceptual model. Front Psychol. 2021;12:635117.
19. Billett S. Critiquing workplace learning discourses: participation and continuity at work. Stud Educ Adults. 2002;34(1):56–67.
20. Eraut M. Informal learning in the workplace. Stud Contin Educ. 2004;26(2):247–73.

21. Billett S. Learning in the workplace: strategies for effective practice [Internet]. 1st ed. Routledge; 2020 [cited 2024 Jun 4]. Available from: https://www.taylorfrancis.com/books/9781000250176
22. Dahl TL, Græslie LS, Petersen SA. Using interactive technology for learning and collaboration to improve organizational culture: a conceptual framework. In: Zaphiris P, Ioannou A, editors. Learning and collaboration technologies: new challenges and learning experiences [Internet], vol. 12784. Cham: Springer; 2021. p. 15–30. [cited 2024 Jun 4] (Lecture Notes in Computer Science). Available from: https://link.springer.com/10.1007/978-3-030-77889-7_2.
23. Dudian M, Abramiuc Todoran T, Popa RA. Organisational culture shifting into online learning. Virtual Learning Practices Stud Bus Econ. 2022;17(3):57–69.
24. Mannion R, Davies H. Understanding organisational culture for healthcare quality improvement. BMJ. 2018:k4907.
25. Li M, Lu C, Yang HH, Wu D, Yang X. The influence of organizational factors on the acceptance of online teaching among college faculty during the COVID-19 pandemic: a nationwide study in mainland China. Educ Technol Res Dev. 2023;71(5):2137–54.
26. Figueiredo AD, Afonso AP. Context and learning: a philosophical framework. In: Figueiredo AD, Afonso AP, editors. Managing learning in virtual settings: the role of context. Hershey, PA: Information Science Publishing; 2006. p. 1–22.
27. Drysdale J. The story is in the structure: a multi-case study of instructional design teams. Online Learn. 2021;25(3):p57–80.
28. Berntz I. Organizational structure types for digital business. Gart Res [Internet]. 2020 Apr 8; Available from: https://www.gartner.com/en/documents/3982139/organizational-structure-types-for-digital-business
29. Çebi A. How e-learning readiness and motivation affect student interactions in distance learning? Educ Inf Technol. 2023;28(3):2941–60.
30. Bandura A, Pastorelli C, Barbaranelli C, Caprara GV. Self-efficacy pathways to childhood depression. J Pers Soc Psychol. 1999;76(2):258.
31. Bandura A. Self-efficacy: toward a unifying theory of behavioral change. Adv Behav Res Ther. 1978;1(4):139–61.
32. Hongsuchon T, Emary IME, Hariguna T, Qhal EMA. Assessing the impact of online-learning effectiveness and benefits in knowledge management, the antecedent of online-learning strategies and motivations: an empirical study. Sustain For. 2022;14(5):2570.
33. McGowin BM, Lockee BB. What's in a name? Defining multimodal environments in higher education. Distance Learn. 2022;19(3):25–38.
34. Rowland P, Anderson M, Kumagai AK, McMillan S, Sandhu VK, Langlois S. Patient involvement in health professionals' education: a meta-narrative review. Adv Health Sci Educ. 2019;24(3):595–617.
35. Bosveld MH, Romme S, De Nooijer J, Smeets HWH, Van Dongen JJJ, Van Bokhoven MA. Seeing the patient as a person in interprofessional health professions education. J Interprof Care. 2023;37(3):457–63.
36. Romme S, Smeets HWH, Bosveld MH, van den Besselaar H, Kline C, Van Bokhoven MA. Involving patients in undergraduate health professions education: what's in it for them? Patient Educ Couns. 2022;105(7):2190–7.
37. Culp J. Educational justice. Philos Compass. 2020;15(12):e12713.

Chapter 4
Best Practice Design and Delivery with Digital Learning Tools

Sathana Dushyanthen, David L. Kok, Alicia Mew, and Michelle Barrett

Abstract This chapter provides a comprehensive guide to creating and implementing cutting-edge digital learning tools for health professional education (HPE). It synthesises the latest research evidence and educational theories for effective digital learning to inform best practices. It examines the pedagogical principles underpinning successful digital education, emphasising the importance of interactivity, engagement, personalisation, and evidence-based content. Key components such as user interface design, accessibility, integration with existing curricula, and evaluation and feedback are discussed in detail. We explore the key drivers behind the integration of technology in HPE and highlight its benefits and challenges. By understanding the context and rationale, educators will gain a solid foundation for designing and delivering effective digital learning experiences. The chapter also offers step-by-step instructions, examples, practical tips, and key considerations for designing and delivering educational content across a variety of digital mediums, including video, graphics, social media, virtual reality (VR), artificial intelligence (AI), podcasts, simulation and gamification. We also delve into the principles of instructional design specifically tailored for HPE, discussing the importance of aligning learning objectives with digital tools and techniques, ensuring that educational content is engaging, interactive, and learner-centred. By presenting practical, evidence-based strategies and showcasing successful implementations, this chapter serves as an invaluable resource for educators, instructional designers, and developers aiming to elevate HPE through innovative digital tools.

S. Dushyanthen
University of Melbourne, Melbourne, VIC, Australia

D. L. Kok (✉)
University of Melbourne, Melbourne, VIC, Australia

Peter MacCallum Cancer Centre, Melbourne, VIC, Australia

Monash University, Melbourne, VIC, Australia
e-mail: dkok@unimelb.edu.au

A. Mew · M. Barrett
Victorian Comprehensive Cancer Centre, Melbourne, VIC, Australia

© The Author(s), under exclusive license to Springer Nature Switzerland AG 2025
D. L. Kok et al. (eds.), *Best Practices in Online Education*, IAMSE Manuals, https://doi.org/10.1007/978-3-031-90349-6_4

Key Points There is a vast array of digital learning tools available to online educators, ranging from video to virtual reality, podcasts, game-based learning and social learning platforms.

- Effective use of these tools requires thoughtful design that aligns pedagogical theory with the educational functionality of each tool.
- There is no single 'right' choice of learning tool for any given educational situation. Choices should be individualised having considered the desired learning outcomes, the alignment between natural strengths of the tool and the topic at hand, available expertise and resourcing, and the overall curricular context.

4.1 Introduction

In recent years, HPE has witnessed a remarkable transformation, due to the rapid advancement of digital technologies. Today, digital learning tools and techniques play a pivotal role in shaping the future of HPE, empowering both educators and learners alike. As medical knowledge expands at an unprecedented pace, educators must adopt best practice design and delivery strategies to harness the potential of digital learning. This chapter guides educators, instructional designers, and medical professionals in designing evidence-based, engaging learning experiences that optimise HPE student learning. We delve into the intricacies of digital learning, exploring cutting-edge tools, techniques, pedagogical principles, and evidence that underpin successful implementation.

We set the stage by examining the evolving landscape of HPE tools and the emergence of digital learning. We explore the key drivers behind the integration of technology in HPE and highlight its benefits and challenges. By understanding the context and rationale, educators will gain a solid foundation for designing and delivering effective digital learning experiences. We also delve into the principles of instructional design specifically tailored for HPE, discussing the importance of aligning learning objectives with digital tools and techniques, ensuring that educational content is engaging, interactive, and learner-centred.

In this chapter, we explore a wide array of digital learning tools that can be harnessed to enhance HPE. Digital learning tools refer to a wide range of software and platforms designed to facilitate and enhance learning in a digital or online environment. They encompass a variety of formats, including websites, apps, software, and delivery modalities, and can serve various educational purposes. From virtual reality (VR) and augmented reality (AR) simulations to physical simulation spaces and mobile applications, this chapter highlights the diverse range of tools available and provides practical insights into their implementation. Through case studies and best practice examples, educators will discover how these tools can be leveraged to create immersive and dynamic learning experiences.

Additionally, we discuss multimedia and the role of audio, video, and interactive graphical media in HPE and the power of visual storytelling, animation, and 3D immersion in conveying complex medical concepts. We also look at how podcasts, as well as polls and quizzes in webinars and online lectures, can enhance the learning experience.

Finally, we focus on online collaboration and social learning in HPE, exploring the importance of creating online communities, fostering peer-to-peer interaction, and promoting collaborative learning using online teamwork tools. We also examine the growing field of artificial intelligence (AI) in HPE, exploring the potential of AI-powered adaptive learning systems, intelligent tutoring systems, and personalised learning algorithms to cater to the unique needs of individual learners. Educators will gain valuable insights into how AI can be integrated into their teaching strategies to optimise learning outcomes. Chapter 7 explores AI in more detail.

We aim to equip educators and medical professionals with the knowledge, skills, and resources needed to navigate the rapidly evolving landscape of digital learning in HPE. By adopting best practice design and delivery strategies, we can create engaging learning opportunities that empower students to take control of their own learning journey and make a memorable impact on their experience.

4.2 Video in HPE

> **Definition** Video in education encompasses a wide range of formats, including recorded lectures, instructional videos, demonstrations, simulated scenarios, interviews, panel discussions, documentaries, animated lessons, and interactive videos.

Video-based learning has emerged as a pivotal tool in HPE, offering a variety of benefits to learners. Research underscores its utility in enhancing retention and understanding, with visual and auditory stimuli working together to foster a deeper comprehension of complex medical subjects [1]. Demonstrations of clinical skills and procedures via videos have been shown to facilitate standardised instruction, allowing students to repeatedly view intricate techniques, thus potentially improving mastery [2]. Additionally, studies have found that video-enhanced simulation and online learning modules, in particular, were linked to positive educational outcomes and, in some cases, outperformed traditional teaching methodologies [2]. Despite these benefits, it is crucial to ensure the quality of video content and its integration with other pedagogical methods to optimise its efficacy in HPE. Studies have shown that video-assisted teaching can enhance the learning experience and improve the acquisition of clinical skills when compared to traditional teaching methods [3]. On another note, embedding questions, quizzes or discussions before viewing videos or within them helps build passive and active viewing. This promotes the cognitive foundation for students to process the information, use critical thinking, as well as explain and clarify amongst each other.

Visual images offer several advantages over verbal communication. Video can:

- Present more information in a given amount of space and time
- Simplify complex concepts
- Clarify pieces of abstract language-based concepts
- Demonstrate concepts/subjects that are in motion and/or relate to one another
- Be more efficient and effective at getting audience attention [2].

For example:

- **Students' Preference**: Many medical students express a preference for video-based resources because they can be replayed, paused, and reviewed at their own pace, catering to individual learning needs.
- **Consistency in Teaching**: Videos can ensure that all students receive the same standard of teaching, which is particularly useful for demonstrating procedures or techniques that require standardisation.

4.2.1 Practical Step-by-Step Instructions for Video Creation [4, 5]

1. **Planning**:
    - Determine the learning objectives of the video and how they relate to the course outcomes.
    - Identify the target audience and their needs.
    - Decide on the style of video (e.g., documentary, panel, interview, piece to camera) (Fig. 4.1)
    - Draft an outline or script and/or storyboard with associated visuals

2. **Production**:
    - Choose a quiet location with good lighting.
    - Use a high-quality camera and microphone.
    - Record the video, ensuring clarity in both visuals and audio.

3. **Editing**:
    - Use video editing software (e.g., Adobe Premiere Pro, Final Cut Pro).
    - Trim unnecessary parts, add annotations, or include supplementary graphics if necessary.
    - Integrate images, concise narration, short annotations, and onscreen captions that are appropriate and relevant.
    - Segment/chunk longer videos into smaller, discrete steps to promote maximal effective use of the audio and visual working memory pathways.

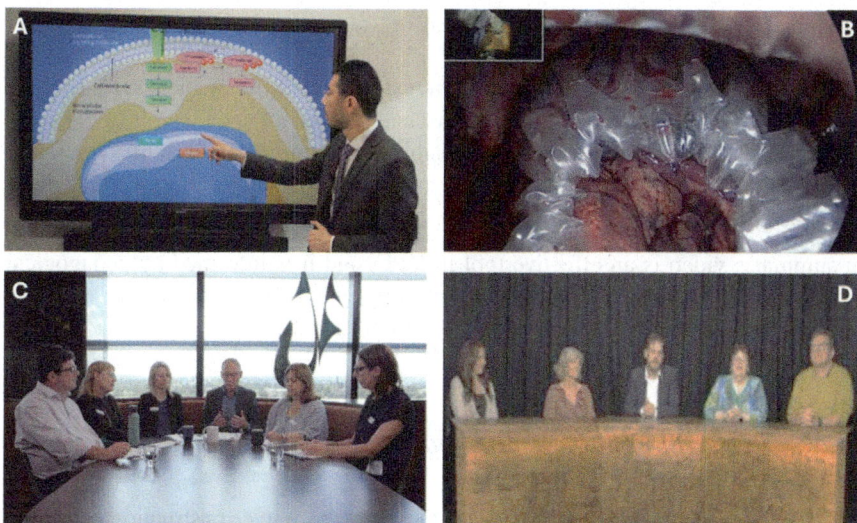

Fig. 4.1 Examples of the types of videos that can be created outside of PowerPoint slides with voiceover. (**a**) Presenter with a touch screen where you can point and highlight different aspects. (**b**) *In situ* demonstrations of procedures with voice-over and annotation. (**c**) Simulated multidisciplinary meeting, round table discussion of real-world patient cases from different perspectives. (**d**) Expert interviews or expert panel with various perspectives represented on a current debate or hot topic

- Consider adding an interactive element every 5 to 10 min to maintain attention and promote participation (e.g., quiz, stop and reflect, discussion, comments).

4. **Review**:

    - Have peers or experts review and provide feedback on the video for accuracy and clarity.

5. **Distribution**:

    - Upload to platforms that are accessible to your target audience (e.g., YouTube, institutional platforms).
    - Review video metrics and analytics to gauge success of deployment, and areas for improvement.

4.2.2 Best-Practice Production and Application [2]

- **Short and Focused**: Keep videos concise. Long videos can overwhelm learners.
- **Interactive Elements**: Include quizzes or interactive elements to engage learners and reinforce learning.

- **High-Quality Visuals and Audio**: Ensure clarity and alignment, as this can greatly affect the learning experience.
- **Incorporate Real-life Scenarios**: Demonstrating real-life medical scenarios can help in bridging the gap between theory and practice.
- **Accessibility**: Ensure videos are accessible to all, considering subtitles for accessibility and ensuring content is clear, appropriately colour-contrasted for those with visual impairments.

In summary, video is an effective tool in HPE, and it is informed by pedagogical theories and empirical research. When creating videos, it is essential to focus on clarity, engagement, and relevance to the learner's needs.

4.2.3 Relevant Pedagogical Theories

- **Constructivist Learning**: Videos can facilitate the active construction of knowledge, allowing learners to integrate new information with their existing knowledge base [6].
- **Multimedia Learning Theory**: this theory posits that people learn more deeply from words and pictures than from words alone. Videos, especially those that combine visual and auditory elements, cater to this principle [7–9] (Fig. 1.2).
- **Cognitive Load Theory**: Well-designed educational videos can manage the cognitive load imposed on learners, ensuring that they are not overwhelmed with information [10, 11].
- **Fractal communication**: "information in a nutshell," served up in modules with five major elements: novelty (contemporary topics), utility (usefulness and timeliness), emotional impact (connection inspiration), conversational (of interest), and entertainment (engaging) [2].
- **Dual-channel principle:** It states that learners can process visual and auditory/written information simultaneously.

See Chap. 1 for detailed descriptions of these relevant learning theories.

4.3 Animation in HPE

> **Definition** Animation in HPE refers to the use of animated visual content to teach and explain medical concepts, procedures and phenomena. This method leverages dynamic visuals and illustrations, often combined with audio explanations.

Animation has emerged as a powerful and effective tool in HPE, offering numerous benefits supported by current evidence. Research studies have shown that animated visuals can enhance the comprehension of complex anatomical structures and physiological processes, aiding in the retention of information and improving students' overall learning experience. Several studies have demonstrated the effectiveness of animations in enhancing learning outcomes and student satisfaction [1]. Additionally, animations can be tailored to illustrate specific medical procedures or pathological conditions, allowing for repeated viewing and practice, which has been linked to increased competence and confidence among learners. Moreover, animation enables educators to simulate dynamic, three-dimensional scenarios, providing a more realistic and engaging learning environment, with the potential to bridge the gap between theory and clinical practice [7, 12]. The growing body of evidence supports the incorporation of animation into medical curricula as an invaluable educational resource, fostering deeper understanding and better-prepared healthcare professionals.

- **Clarification of complex topics**: Animations can simplify intricate processes, such as cellular mechanisms or biochemical pathways, making them easier to comprehend.
- **Engagement & motivation**: Animated content tends to be more engaging than static images or text, potentially leading to better motivation and retention (Table. 4.1).

Table 4.1 Evidence-based multimedia learning principles (adapted from Yue et al. [13] and Mayer [14])

Learning principle	Definition	Recommendations
Managing essential processing		
Pre-training principle	Relevant information presented before the animation to allow learners to familiarise before having to work with something increases learning efficiency.	Provide a glossary of key terms, basic definitions or concepts that will be used in the animation.
Modality principle	Words accompanying an animation are presented orally instead of visually.	Present spoken text to augment visual content so learners can listen and refer to graphic. Limit text used.
Segmenting principle	Learning is best when information is presented in segments, rather than one long continuous stream.	Add self-paced options to enable learners to process information before continuing. Chunk longer videos into smaller bit-sized pieces. Consider chapterisation.
Multimedia principle	People learn better from words and pictures than from words alone.	Use relevant graphics and narration, rather than text on screen and audio voice over.
Minimising extraneous processing		
Coherence principle	Animation contains only educationally relevant pictorial and verbal information.	Eliminate background music, unrelated or unnecessarily flashy graphics, even if they appear interesting, as this reduces cognitive capacity to process essential information. Less is more.

(continued)

Table 4.1 (continued)

Learning principle	Definition	Recommendations
Redundancy principle	Learning is best with narration and graphics, as opposed to narration, graphics, and text (i.e.. on-screen text does not duplicate narration)	Rely on narration to communicate verbal information. If on-screen text must be used, present as labels or 1–2 key words rather than sentences.
Signalling principle	Learning is best when learners are shown exactly what to pay attention to on the screen. Cues prompt learners to the organisation of essential material.	Prior to the animation, provide an outline of the content. If the animation describes steps, list them all first before repeating and elaborating on each one. Show the learner what exactly to pay attention to through highlighting, circling, enlarging etc.
Temporal contiguity principle	Visual elements are synchronised with corresponding narration, words placed near graphics.	Synchronise the timing of the animation with corresponding words in the narration
Spatial contiguity principle	Labels are placed close to visual elements	Place labels on or next to associated images, use arrow and connectors to link text to graphic
Facilitating generative processing		
Interactivity principle	Learners control the order, pace and other interactive elements of the animation.	Allow learners to pause, navigate through different segments of the animation, and manipulate parameters (e.g., rotate body part, zoom in/out).
Personalisation principle	Learning is best from a more informal, conversational voice than an overly formal voice. Having a more casual voice actually improves the learning experience.	Present words in conversational style rather than formal style.
Voice principle	Learning is best from human voice, rather than a computer voice.	Use narration with personable, clear human voice, rather than computer or AI generated voice, which matches visuals.
Image principle	Do not necessarily learn better from a multimedia lesson when the speaker's image is added to the screen.	Instead of a talking head, use graphics that illustrate the narration.
Embodiment principle	Learn more deeply when on-screen agents display humanlike gesturing, movement, eye contact, and facial expressions rather than not.	Drawing graphics as you explain is more beneficial than explaining a presented drawing.

Animations should be designed with the learner's cognitive capacity in mind and aim to optimise the balance among three types of cognitive demand: essential processing, extraneous processing, and generative processing

4.3.1 Practical Step-by-Step Instructions for Animation Creation:

1. **Planning**:
   - Determine the objectives of the animation.
   - Draft an outline or storyboard detailing the progression of the animation.
   - Decide on animation style (e.g., doodle, 2D, 3D, stock footage) (Fig. 4.2).

2. **Design**:
   - Design characters, symbols, and other elements. Consider using a consistent colour palette and style.

3. **Animation**:
   - Use animation software (e.g., Adobe Animate, Blender).
   - Animate the characters and elements according to your storyboard.
   - Add voiceovers or background music as needed.

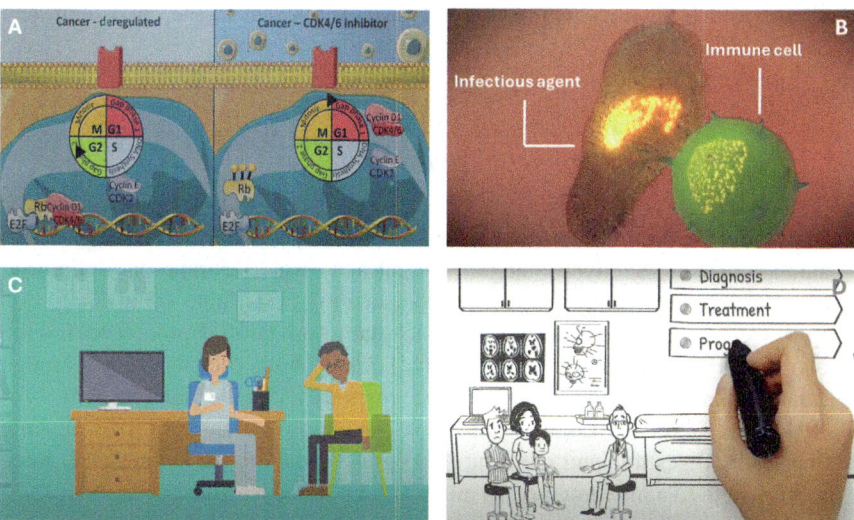

Fig. 4.2 Examples of different types of animations that can be used in HPE. (**a**) 2D molecular signalling processes. (**b**) 3D cellular processes, (**c**) 2D character depictions of clinical scenarios. (**d**) 2D doodle drawing of medical processes. (Stills are taken from videos produced by our team and are also available on Science in Motion and YouTube.)

4. **Editing**:
   - Fine-tune the animation, ensuring synchronisation between audio and visual elements.

5. **Review**:
   - Peer or expert review is crucial for ensuring accuracy and clarity in medical content.

6. **Distribution**:
   - Publish on platforms accessible to your target audience, considering proprietary platforms for educational institutions or public platforms like YouTube.

4.3.2 Best-Practice Production and Application:

- **Keep It Simple**: Avoid overloading the animation with too much information.
- **Narration**: A clear voiceover can guide learners through the animation, reinforcing concepts.
- **Interactivity**: Consider adding interactive elements or quizzes post-animation to reinforce learning.
- **High-Quality Design**: Clear, professional visuals and audio can make a significant difference in the learner's experience.
- **Contextual Relevance**: Ensure animations are relevant to the curriculum and contextualised to real-life medical scenarios when possible.

4.3.3 Relevant Pedagogical Theories

- **Cognitive Theory of Multimedia Learning (CTML)**: This theory suggests that animations can effectively integrate verbal and visual information, optimising cognitive processing and deepening understanding [13] (Table 1.3 in Chap. 1).
- **Dual Coding Theory:** This theory posits that information is processed through two distinct channels (visual and verbal). Using both channels (e.g., through animations with voiceovers) can enhance memory and understanding [15].
- **Reducing Cognitive Load:** Animations can simplify complex topics, making them more digestible and reducing the cognitive load on the learner [13]. Keep video length to a maximum of 10 minutes. Chunk longer videos.
- **Active processing:** Learners engage in active learning by attending to relevant incoming information, organising selected information into coherent mental representations, and integrating mental representation with other knowledge.

See Chap. 1 for detailed descriptions of these relevant learning theories.

In conclusion, animations have proven to be an effective tool in HPE, both from research outcomes and pedagogical perspectives. When producing animations, ensuring clarity, relevance, and engagement is vital for optimal learning outcomes.

4.4 Graphics and Infographics in HPE

> **Definition** Infographics and graphics in HPE refer to visual representations of medical information designed to simplify and clarify complex data and concepts. These graphics combine text, images, and design elements to communicate information quickly and effectively in an engaging manner.

The integration of graphics and infographics into HPE has gained prominence due to the compelling evidence of their effectiveness. Research has shown that visual aids, such as infographics, enhance the comprehension of complex medical concepts and facilitate information retention among learners. Graphics and infographics can efficiently convey intricate anatomical structures, disease pathways, and pharmacological mechanisms, making them particularly valuable for simplifying and visualising intricate medical information. Furthermore, the interactive nature of infographics encourages active learning and critical thinking, enabling students to process and synthesise information effectively. This growing body of evidence highlights the potential of graphics and infographics as essential tools in HPE, offering a visually engaging and pedagogically sound approach to knowledge dissemination [16].

- **Research Outcomes**: Visual aids, such as infographics, have demonstrated their effectiveness in enhancing understanding and retention, noting the value of visual aids, including infographics, in HPE.
- **Enhancing Memory**: Infographics can promote recall by leveraging visual memory, highlighting the advantage of using both visual and verbal cues to promote memory.
- **Complexity Simplification**: Medical science and medicine often involve intricate concepts. Infographics can break down these ideas into more digestible formats, aiding understanding.

Figure 4.3 illustrates two examples of the use of graphics and infographics in HPE.

4.4.1 Practical Step-by-Step Instructions for Infographic Creation:

1. **Planning**:
    - Determine the objectives and target audience.
    - Decide on the main points to communicate.
    - Draft an outline or a rough sketch.

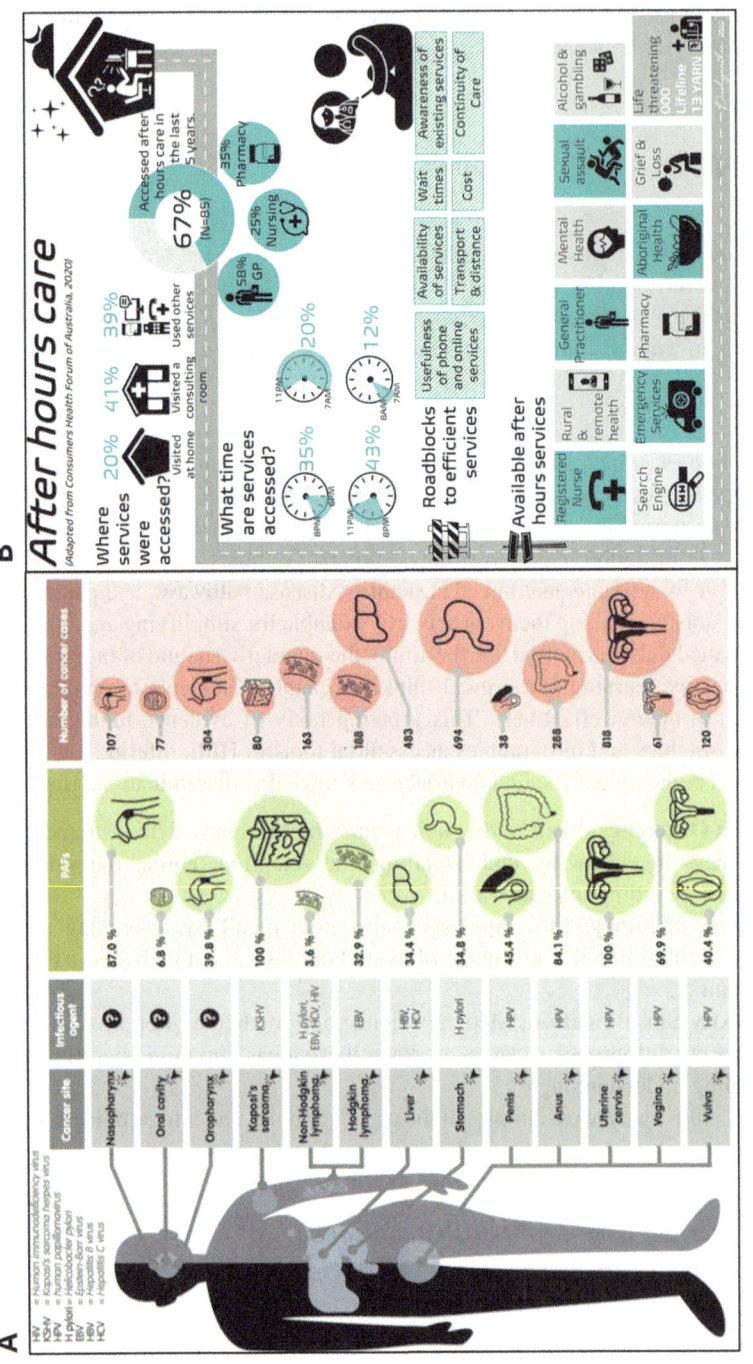

Fig. 4.3 Examples of (**a**) graphics [17] and (**b**) infographics that can be used in HPE [18]. (**a**) example of an interactive graphic that demonstrates the population attributable fraction (PAF) and data on cancer incidence by cancer site and infectious agent. It contains clickable elements and circles are proportional. (**b**) Represents a static infographic that presents information and statistics for after-hours care options

2. **Design**:
   - Choose a layout: vertical, horizontal, or matrix.
   - Use a consistent colour scheme, preferably one that resonates with the topic.
   - Use icons, symbols, and other visuals that align with the content.
3. **Creation**:
   - Use graphic design software (e.g., Adobe Illustrator, Canva).
   - Integrate visuals and text. Ensure a balanced layout.
4. **Editing & Review**:
   - Proofread for any typos or inaccuracies.
   - Ensure clarity and coherence.
   - Seek feedback from peers or experts in the field.
5. **Distribution**:
   - Share on the desired platforms, be it print, online platforms, or within educational materials (Fig. 4.3).

4.4.2 Best-Practice Production and Application

- **Clarity is key**: The main objective of an infographic is to convey information clearly. Avoid clutter.
- **Hierarchy**: Ensure that the most important information is the most prominent, using size, colour, and positioning (Fig. 4.4).
- **Cite sources**: In a field like medicine, accuracy is crucial. Always cite your sources.
- **Interactivity**: When used online, interactive infographics can enhance engagement.
- **Accessibility**: Ensure that graphics are accessible to all, considering colour blindness and ensuring content is clear for those with visual impairments.

4.4.3 Relevant Pedagogical Theories

- **Dual Coding Theory**: using both verbal and visual information can aid in memory and understanding. Infographics cater to this by combining text with imagery.
- **Cognitive Load Theory**: Graphics can streamline information, reducing the cognitive load and making learning more efficient.
- **Constructivist Learning**: Infographics can provide scaffolds upon which learners can construct knowledge, integrating new information with prior understanding.

See Chap. 1 for detailed descriptions of these relevant learning theories.

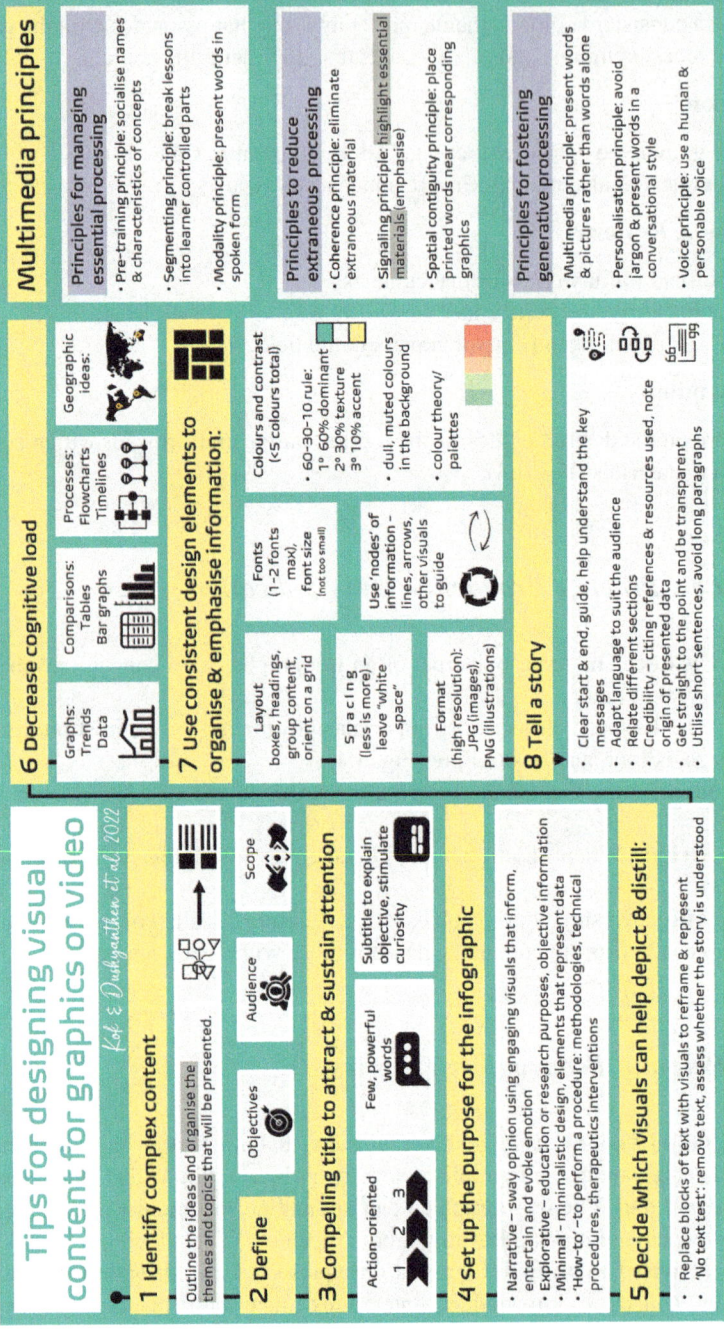

Fig. 4.4 Tips, steps and multimedia principles for designing visuals for text or video [18]

To conclude, graphics and infographics in HPE can be immensely beneficial, backed by both empirical research and pedagogical theories. Effective design, which is clear and engaging, is at the heart of maximising the benefits of these visual tools.

4.5 Social Learning Tools in HPE

> **Definition** Social learning tools in HPE refer to digital platforms and technologies that facilitate collaborative learning, knowledge sharing, and peer interaction among students, professionals, and educators. These tools leverage social networking, communication, and collaborative features to enhance the educational experience.

The adoption of social learning tools in HPE has garnered substantial attention, supported by a growing body of evidence affirming their efficacy. Studies have demonstrated that social learning platforms, such as online discussion forums and collaborative learning environments, enhance student engagement, foster peer-to-peer interaction, and promote the exchange of knowledge and experiences, which are essential components of HPE. Moreover, these tools facilitate the development of critical thinking and problem-solving skills by encouraging active participation and the exploration of diverse perspectives. Research has also highlighted the role of social learning in reducing learner isolation, enhancing motivation, and improving overall academic performance, suggesting that they hold significant promise in preparing healthcare professionals for the complex challenges they will encounter in their careers. The accumulating evidence underscores the value of integrating social learning tools into HPE to nurture collaborative and reflective practitioners [19–22].

4.5.1 Practical Step-by-Step Instructions for Incorporating Social Learning Tools:

1. **Objectives & Planning**:
   - Define the learning objectives and outcomes.
   - Determine the most appropriate tool(s) for the purpose.
2. **Selection of Tool**:
   - Discussion Platforms: Slack, Microsoft Teams, or built-in forums on Learning Management Systems like Moodle or Blackboard.

- Collaborative Platforms: MS Teams, Google Docs, Wikis, Trello.
- Social Media Platforms: Twitter (for academic discussions using hashtags), Facebook groups, or LinkedIn groups (Table 4.2).

3. **Setup & Customisation**:
   - Customise the platform: Ensure privacy settings are appropriate, especially given the sensitive nature of medical information.
   - Structure: Create specific channels or threads for various topics or modules.

4. **Integration**:
   - Embed relevant resources, readings, or other educational materials.
   - Provide guidelines or tutorials on how to use the platform.

Table 4.2 Social learning platforms commonly used in higher education, along with their descriptions

Platform	Description
Moodle/Canvas/Blackboard (Learning Management System)	Learning management system with features such as discussion boards, wikis, quizzes, HTML embed, group projects, and peer reviews to promote interaction and collaboration among students.
Microsoft Teams	Collaboration platform with chat, video meetings, and integration with Office 365, facilitating group work and communication among students and faculty through shared documents.
Slack	Messaging app for team collaboration that supports channels for different topics, direct messaging, file sharing, and integration with other tools.
Google Classroom	Education-focused platform that simplifies creating, distributing, and grading assignments while supporting collaboration through Google Workspace tools.
Yammer	Enterprise social networking service by Microsoft that enables communication and collaboration within educational institutions and among student groups.
Padlet	Online bulletin board for collaboration, where students and teachers can post notes, images, links, and documents for group projects and discussions.
Kahoot!, Mentimeter, PollEv, Slido	Game-based learning platform that creates interactive quizzes and challenges, promoting engagement and friendly competition among students.
Trello	Project management tool that supports collaborative planning and task management through boards, lists, and cards, useful for group projects and assignments.
Miro, Mural, Jamboard, Figma, Mindmeister, MS whiteboard	Online collaborative whiteboard platform for brainstorming, planning, and teamwork, allowing students to work together in real-time.
Discord	Communication platform with text, voice, and video capabilities, popular for creating study groups and class communities where students can collaborate and share.

5. **Engagement & Moderation**:
   - Initiate discussions or collaborative tasks.
   - Assign educators or experienced students as moderators to ensure constructive discussions and correct any misconceptions.
6. **Feedback & Iteration**:
   - Periodically solicit feedback from students.
   - Adapt and modify based on feedback and evolving needs.

4.5.2 Best-Practice Production and Application

- **Clear Guidelines**: Establish clear communication and behaviour guidelines from the onset.
- **Privacy & Security**: Given that medical discussions can include sensitive or identifiable patient data and student's personal information, ensure that platforms are secure and users are educated about maintaining confidentiality.
- **Blended Approach**: Combine social learning tools with traditional teaching methods for a comprehensive learning experience.
- **Diverse Formats**: Use a mix of text, video, quizzes, and other interactive elements to cater to different learning styles and needs.
- **Ongoing Engagement**: Regularly update content and engage with students to keep the platform lively and beneficial.

4.5.3 Relevant Pedagogical Theories

Social Constructivism: Rooted in the work of **Vygotsky**, this theory posits that learning is a socially mediated activity. Interactive tools can foster this by allowing students to collaborate, discuss, and construct knowledge together [22].

Connectivism: **Siemens (2005)** emphasises the importance of networks, connections, and technology in contemporary learning. Social learning tools embody this by facilitating connections, discussions, and shared resources [23].

Communities of Practice: **Wenger (1998)** highlighted that learning is deeply social and often occurs in communities centered around shared practices or interests. Social learning tools can help form and sustain these communities [24].

See Chap. 1 for detailed descriptions of these relevant learning theories.

In summary, social learning tools present immense potential in HPE, as evidenced by research and backed by various pedagogical theories. Effective utilisation requires careful planning, setup, and moderation to ensure they are used constructively and safely.

4.6 Virtual Reality and Augmented Reality in HPE

> **Definition** Augmented Reality (AR) refers to the integration of digital information with the user's environment in real time. In HPE, AR overlays digital content, such as images, videos, and 3D models, onto the physical world. Virtual Reality (VR) is a fully immersive digital environment where users can interact with 3D models and scenarios using VR headsets and controllers. In HPE, VR creates realistic simulations of medical environments, procedures, and scenarios.

The utilisation of VR and AR in HPE has gained considerable momentum, underpinned by a growing body of evidence that underscores their transformative potential. VR technology creates entirely artificial environments through headsets that isolate users from their surroundings. In comparison, AR overlays digital interfaces upon physical surroundings, producing an environment that is both real and digital [25]. Research has revealed that VR and AR technologies can enhance medical training by providing immersive, three-dimensional simulations for anatomy and surgical procedures, and radiotherapy training [26], offering a safe and repeatable environment for skill development [27]. These technologies also enable students to explore and manipulate anatomical structures in ways that were previously unattainable, promoting better understanding and retention of complex information. On another note, VR can also be used for therapy and patient education, such as to treat phobias, post-traumatic stress disorder (PTSD), rehabilitation and pain management [26]. AR, in particular, has shown promise in real-time medical imaging and clinical decision support, assisting students and professionals in diagnosing and treating patients more effectively [28]. The evidence suggests that VR and AR have the potential to revolutionise HPE, bridging the gap between theory and practice and fostering a new era of highly skilled and clinically competent healthcare practitioners [29–31].

4.6.1 Practical Step-by-Step Instructions for Virtual Reality and Augmented Reality Creation:

1. **Planning & Objectives**:
    - Determine the learning outcomes.
    - Decide on scenarios or procedures to simulate.
2. **Design & Storyboarding**:
    - Design the virtual environment or augmented overlay.
    - Storyboard sequences, especially if simulating procedures.
    - Script dialogues between patients and clinicians.

3. **Tool Selection**:
   - Choose appropriate software: Unity, and Unreal Engine for VR/AR development.
   - Decide on hardware: Oculus Rift, HTC (High Tech Computer Corporation) Vive for VR; Microsoft HoloLens for AR.

4. **Development**:
   - Develop the environment using the chosen software.
   - Incorporate interactive elements, open text or multiple-choice questions, feedback mechanisms, and scoring (if applicable).

5. **Testing**:
   - Pilot the VR/AR experience with a group of learners.
   - Collect feedback on usability, realism, and educational value.

6. **Deployment**:
   - Integrate into the curriculum.
   - Ensure the availability of necessary VR/AR hardware for learners.

4.6.2 Best-Practice Production and Application:

- **Realism**: Ensure the virtual environment is as realistic as possible to enhance the learning experience.
- **Interactivity**: Engage learners through tasks, feedback, and decision-making within the virtual environment.
- **Safety & Comfort**: Ensure VR/AR experiences don't cause motion sickness or discomfort. Provide breaks during longer sessions.
- **Debriefing**: After a VR/AR session, engage learners in discussions or reflections to consolidate learning.
- **Blended Approach**: Combine VR/AR experiences with traditional teaching methods and other technological tools for a comprehensive learning experience.

4.6.3 Relevant Pedagogical Theories

- **Experiential Learning**: Rooted in **Kolb's (1984)** work, this theory underscores the value of direct experience in the learning process. VR and AR offer immersive experiences, allowing students to practice in controlled, virtual environments [22] (Fig. 4.5).

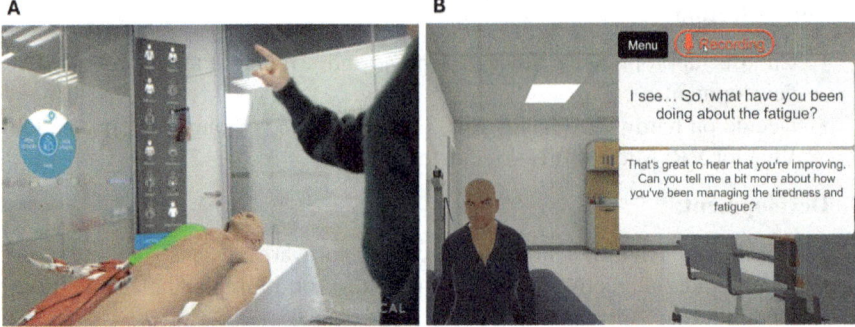

Fig. 4.5 Examples of (**a**) augmented reality and (**b**) virtual reality in HPE. (**a**) The AR app 'HoloHuman' displays a virtual cadaver, projected on a real-world space. The learner can interact with the model and user interface through the use of a HoloLens headset. Structures, organs and systems can be examined, supported by visual narratives and digital dissection tools (3D4 Medical from Elsevier, 2020) [31]. (**b**) Fully immersive VR environment exploring communication skills between patients and clinicians [32]. Reproduced under CC BY 4.0

- **Situated Learning**: **Lave & Wenger (1991)** emphasised learning as a process of participation in communities of practice. VR and AR can simulate real-world clinical settings, thus situating learning in practice-based contexts [22].
- **Cognitive Load Theory**: VR and AR can streamline complex information, offering layered, interactive experiences that can be tailored to manage cognitive load [14].

See Chap. 1 for detailed descriptions of these relevant learning theories.

In conclusion, VR and AR in HPE offer transformative experiences, allowing students to immerse themselves in virtual clinical settings, improving both skills and knowledge. Their adoption is supported by several pedagogical theories, emphasising the importance of situated and experiential learning. Proper planning, development, and application are crucial for harnessing the full potential of these technologies.

4.7 Simulation in HPE

Definition Simulation in HPE refers to the use of advanced techniques and technologies (e.g. mannequin-based (nowadays commonly referred to as manikins), patient actors, virtual simulation, task trainer, or some hybrid form of these technologies) to create realistic, interactive scenarios that mimic clinical situations for the purpose of training healthcare professionals. These simulations provide a safe and controlled environment for students and professionals to practice skills, make decisions, and experience the consequences of their actions without risking patient safety.

The integration of simulations, whether it is for skill or scenario-based learning (SBL) in HPE, has been substantiated by a wealth of evidence showcasing their effectiveness. Research demonstrates that medical simulations, including high-fidelity manikins, virtual patient scenarios, and task trainers, are invaluable tools for teaching and assessing clinical skills, improving decision-making, and enhancing overall competency among medical learners [33]. Some common applications of SBL include supporting patient safety and quality programmes, skills training and competency assessment, ameliorating clinical teaching constraints, and supporting the development of interprofessional collaborative practice [33]. Simulations allow students to practice a wide range of procedures and complex medical scenarios in a safe and controlled environment, reducing the risk to real patients. They promote active learning, teamwork, and the development of problem-solving skills by engaging students in realistic clinical situations [34]. As a result, the use of simulations has become integral in HPE, offering a bridge between theoretical knowledge and practical application and ultimately better preparing future healthcare professionals.

4.7.1 Practical Step-by-Step Instructions for Simulation Creation:

1. **Needs Assessment**:
   - Define the learning objectives and determine what skills or situations need to be addressed (Table 4.3).
2. **Design**:
   - Storyboard scenarios.
   - Choose the type of simulation: mannequin-based, computer-based, standardised patients, escape room, or task trainers.
3. **Development**:
   - Create or purchase the necessary equipment or software.
   - Script scenarios, potentially with branching decisions.
4. **Training**:
   - Train facilitators and standardised patients, if used.
   - Ensure facilitators understand debriefing techniques.
5. **Implementation**:
   - Set up the simulation environment.
   - Brief participants on the objectives and format.

Table 4.3 Simulation principles (adapted from Lopreiato and Sawyer [33])

Principle	Description	Example
Curriculum integration	Integrating simulation as part of the overall curricular plan to include clear learning objectives	A septic shock simulation is included as part of the emergency medicine rotation to reinforce diagnosis and treatment of septic shock.
Feedback and debriefing	Including a structured debriefing immediately after a simulation, conducted using an accepted approach which ensures the psychological safety of the participants	After a simulated cardiac arrest scenario, the residents are lead through a facilitated discussion of what occurred during the simulation. Feedback on ways performance could be improved in the future is provided.
Deliberate practice	Allowing residents the ability to practice a procedural skill with directed feedback until they are proficient	Residents participated in an airway skills training session where they are allowed to intubate a task trainer repeatedly while receiving directive feedback on their performance.
Mastery learning	Practicing a skill to a level where coaching is not necessary, and performance has achieved a mastery level	During an airway skills session, residents undergo baseline testing before receiving standardised instruction and deliberate practice with focused feedback. After significant deliberate practice the residents undergo a post-test to confirm performance at a predefined mastery level using a valid and reliable airway skills assessment tool.
Range of difficulty and clinical variation	Varying the complexity of simulation scenarios on the basis of the year group of residents involved and including a variety of problems to be solved in a scenario	During the course of residency, residents participate in simulation of escalating intensity and difficulty as they progress from first, second to third year. Additionally, after proficiency is attained in one scenario, the scenario is changed to avoid repetition and monotony.

6. **Debriefing**:
    - After the simulation, discuss the participants' actions, decisions, and thought processes.
    - Emphasise reflective learning and constructive feedback.
7. **Evaluation & Feedback**:
    - Assess participant performance.
    - Collect feedback to improve the simulation.

4.7.2 Best-Practice Production and Application [35]

- **Fidelity**: While high-fidelity simulations can be immersive, fidelity should match the learning objectives. Sometimes, low-fidelity simulations can be equally effective.

- **Safe Environment**: Ensure that the simulation environment feels psychologically safe, promoting open discussion and learning.
- **Repetitive Practice**: Allow learners to practice multiple times, refining their skills with each iteration.
- **Debriefing**: This is a crucial phase where most of the reflective learning happens. The facilitator plays a vital role in guiding this discussion.
- **Integration**: Simulation should be integrated into the broader curriculum, linking it to theoretical knowledge and real clinical experiences.
- **Variability**: Expose learners to a variety of cases and situations to improve their adaptability and generalisability of skills.

4.7.3 Relevant Pedagogical Theories

- **Experiential Learning**: **Kolb (1984)** posited that learning is a process whereby knowledge is created through the transformation of experience. Simulation provides a controlled environment for such experiences [22].
- **Situated Cognition**: This theory suggests that learning often happens best when it's rooted in authentic contexts and activities. Simulations offer these "authentic" environments [36, 37].
- **Deliberate Practice**: **Ericsson, K. A. (2004)** discussed the role of deliberate and repeated practice in achieving expertise. Simulation allows for this repeated, focused practice [38, 39].

See Chap. 1 for detailed descriptions of these relevant learning theories.

In conclusion, simulation-based HPE, grounded in strong pedagogical foundations, offers a controlled and safe environment for learners to practice and refine their skills. Its effectiveness is well-documented, and its implementation requires careful planning, development, and facilitation to achieve the desired outcomes.

4.8 Podcasts in HPE

> **Definition** Podcasts in HPE are audio programs that cover a wide range of medical topics, such as interviews, lectures, case studies, discussions, and updates on the latest research and clinical practices.

Podcasts have gained recognition as a valuable resource in HPE, supported by a growing body of evidence highlighting their effectiveness. Research has shown that podcasts offer flexibility and accessibility for learners, enabling them to engage with educational content at their own pace and convenience [40]. Listeners have identified podcasts as a more efficient and enjoyable way to keep up to date [41].

Second, podcasting offers exposure to international expertise that may not otherwise be accessible. Third, the format creates a low-stress atmosphere that is less intimidating to learners. Podcasts create low-stakes dialogue that engenders a positive learning environment [40]. They are particularly beneficial for delivering complex medical topics, clinical case discussions, and expert interviews, enhancing content retention and knowledge acquisition. Moreover, the use of podcasts can serve as a complementary tool for traditional teaching methods, contributing to a more comprehensive and engaging learning experience in both undergraduate and postgraduate HPE. Many of the more popular HPE podcasts offer a casual tone and "show notes" that offer visual summaries of topics discussed or links to enable learners to find primary sources mentioned [42]. Podcasts are virtual communities of practice. Unlike one's static institutional environment, podcasts offer learners an opportunity to tune in to the community of practice of their choosing. The available evidence underscores the potential of podcasts as a dynamic and user-friendly medium for disseminating medical knowledge [43].

4.8.1 Practical Step-by-Step Instructions for Podcast Creation [41]

1. **Planning & Content Design**:
    - Define the topic, objectives, and target audience.
    - Research and gather necessary content and citations and ensure the accuracy of information.
    - Create a rough script or outline to ensure flow. It should sound natural.
    - Provide guests with a rough guide of the questions prior to the podcast to avoid misquotes and going off track, and allow time for preparation.
    - The "host" should be knowledgeable in the area and lively and engaging.

2. **Recording**:
    - Use a good-quality microphone for clear audio.
    - Choose a quiet environment to minimise background noise.
    - Use recording software like Audacity, GarageBand, or Adobe Audition.

3. **Editing**:
    - Remove unnecessary pauses, "ums", and "uhs".
    - Remove background noise.
    - Add intro and outro (concluding section of a piece of media) music, if desired. Ensure you have the right to use any music.

4. **Publishing**:
    - Choose a podcast hosting platform: Apple, Spotify, local website, LMS.
    - Create a catchy title, description, and cover art.

5. **Promotion**:
    - Share on social media, medical forums, and within institutional channels.
    - Encourage feedback and reviews to improve.

4.8.2 Best-Practice Production and Application

- **Relevance**: Ensure the content is current and relevant to the audience. This is crucial in HPE, where outdated information can have serious implications.
- **Duration**: Medical students and professionals often have tight schedules. It is best to keep podcasts concise and focused. Generally, 20–30 min is a sweet spot. A long recording that covers a broad topic can also be edited and released as 'parts' based on subtopics to reduce individual episode length.
- **Engagement**: Use case discussions, interviews, and narratives to keep the audience engaged. Avoid monotonous lectures.
- **Accessibility**: Make podcasts easily accessible on various platforms such as Apple Podcasts, Spotify, Google Podcasts, and LMS.
- **Regular Updates**: If creating a series, ensure regular updates to maintain listener engagement and provide ongoing value.
- **Feedback Loop**: Encourage listeners to provide feedback. This can inform improvements and ensure the podcast meets learners' needs.

4.8.3 Relevant Pedagogical Theories [22]

- **Constructivism**: Podcasts, especially those that employ narratives or case discussions, align with the idea that learning is an active, constructive process. Learners interpret podcast content based on their prior knowledge.
- **Self-directed Learning/Andragogy**: Podcasts empower learners to take control of their learning, choosing when, where, and how they engage with content.
- **Multimodal Learning**: Podcasts appeal to auditory learners and can complement visual and kinesthetic learning (e.g. physical activities, hands-on experiences, and movement) modes.
- **Social learning theory:** Individuals learn by observing others; listening to others may not only disseminate medical knowledge but also engage in critical thinking and sharing cultural competencies.

See Chap. 1 for detailed descriptions of these relevant learning theories.

In conclusion, podcasts offer a versatile and modern approach to HPE, enabling learners to consume content at their own pace and convenience. Their effectiveness, supported by pedagogical theories, makes them an invaluable tool for educators. Proper planning, production, and continuous engagement with the audience are key to a successful podcast in HPE.

4.9 Branched Scenarios in HPE

> **Definition** Branched scenarios in HPE are interactive, case-based learning tools that allow learners to make decisions at key points in a clinical scenario, leading to different outcomes based on their choices.

The use of branched scenarios in HPE has emerged as a promising and evidence-backed pedagogical approach. Research has indicated that branched scenarios, where learners make decisions that lead to different outcomes, foster critical thinking, clinical reasoning, and decision-making skills essential for healthcare professionals. This interactive format encourages active engagement and provides a safe space for learners to make and learn from mistakes, enhancing their competence and confidence. Furthermore, branched scenarios have been particularly effective in training healthcare practitioners to manage complex and dynamic clinical situations, offering an active and adaptive learning experience. The current evidence underscores the value of branched scenarios as an innovative and impactful method for HPE, facilitating the development of clinical expertise and the ability to navigate real-world healthcare challenges [44].

4.9.1 Practical Step-by-Step Instructions for Branched Scenario Creation

1. **Define Objectives**:
   - Identify what you want learners to understand or be able to do after completing the scenario.
2. **Draft a Narrative**:
   - Create a storyline, ideally based on real-life situations or cases.
3. **Decide on Branch Points**:
   - Determine critical decision points within the narrative where learners must choose a path.
4. **Develop Outcomes**:
   - For each decision point, create outcomes or consequences. Some can lead to further decisions, while others might conclude the scenario.
5. **Choose a Platform/Tool**:
   - Use tools like Twine, H5P, BranchTrack, or even PowerPoint to build your scenario.

6. **Design & Build**:
   - Incorporate multimedia elements (images, audio) if relevant.
   - Ensure a clear and intuitive user interface.
7. **Test & Refine**:
   - Have peers and target learners test the scenario.
   - Revise based on feedback.

4.9.2 Best-Practice Production and Application

- **Realism**: Scenarios should be authentic, representing real-world situations medical learners might face.
- **Feedback**: Provide learners with feedback on their decisions, explaining why certain choices were correct or incorrect.
- **Multiple Paths**: Allow multiple pathways to success. In medicine, there may be more than one right answer or approach.
- **Accessibility**: Ensure that branched scenarios are accessible on various devices, considering mobile compatibility.
- **Integration**: Incorporate scenarios within broader curricula, connecting them to lectures, readings, and other learning resources.

4.9.3 Relevant Pedagogical Theories

- **Constructivism**: Branched scenarios align with constructivist principles, allowing learners to construct knowledge through interactions within a virtual environment [22].
- **Situated Learning**: Scenarios provide contextualised learning experiences, offering a "situated" environment where learners can practice and apply knowledge.
- **Experiential Learning: Kolb's** theory emphasises learning through reflection on doing, which branched scenarios facilitate by allowing learners to make decisions and reflect upon the outcomes [22].

See Chap. 1 for detailed descriptions of these relevant learning theories.

In conclusion, branched scenarios provide an interactive and engaging method for medical learners to hone their decision-making skills in a risk-free environment. Their efficacy, grounded in pedagogical theories like constructivism and experiential learning, makes them a valuable tool in HPE. Proper design, integration, and regular updates ensure that they remain relevant and effective for learners.

4.10 Game-Based Learning in HPE

> **Definition** Gamification in HPE refers to the application of interactive and immersive game design elements, principles and activities by incorporating aspects such as points, badges, leaderboards, challenges, and interactive storytelling to teach medical concepts, skills, and decision-making processes.

Game-based learning and gamification are increasingly recognised as effective strategies in HPE, supported by a growing body of evidence. Research has shown that these approaches enhance student engagement, motivation, and knowledge retention by providing an interactive and enjoyable learning experience with immediate feedback [45]. Games and gamified content in HPE offer opportunities for students to practice clinical decision-making, critical thinking, and problem-solving in a risk-free environment, which is particularly valuable for preparing them for real-world healthcare scenarios [45, 46]. Additionally, the use of leaderboards, badges, and rewards has been associated with increased participation and competition, fostering a sense of achievement and progression among learners [47]. The current evidence underscores the effectiveness of game-based learning and gamification in HPE as innovative tools for enhancing student performance and motivation [44].

4.10.1 Practical Step-by-Step Instructions for Game Creation

1. **Define Objectives**:
   - What should learners understand or be able to do after playing the game?
2. **Conceptualise the Game**:
   - Will it be a board game, digital game, or simulation?
   - Decide on game mechanics: point scoring, competition, role-playing, Q&A, quiz etc.
3. **Design & Develop**:
   - Outline game rules, challenges, and rewards (Table 4.4).
   - For digital games, choose a platform or game engine (e.g., Unity, Unreal Engine).
   - Incorporate educational content seamlessly.
4. **Test**:
   - Pilot the game with a small group of learners.
   - Gather feedback on gameplay, educational content, and user experience.

Table 4.4 Principles for scenario or game design (adapted from Argueta-Munoz et al. [44])

Components	Description
Target population	Define the population to which the game is directed and recognise its characteristics (academic degree, use of technology, information management).
Objectives	Define the general and specific objectives. Define learning outcomes. Design the rules and the way components of the game interact. Consider that the decision-making points are clear, easily identifiable, and attached to the game's objective.
Game features	Establish components, characters or avatars and the environment in which it takes place. Determine the usability; how easy it is to use. Consider how easy it will be to access the game. Test the integration and the interactions of the game elements. Define the website or where the game will be stored and distributed. Set whether the game is multiplayer or single player. Set the number of levels and methods to access them. Define the relationship between the users. Communication between peers, superiors, or cognitive aids to advance within the story. Write clear and precise rules for how components, characters, players, and environment interact during development. The system of rewards and penalties and save points will have to be specified.
Programming design tool	Consider the graphics and requirements and what tool will be required (e.g. Unity, Blender). What skills and expertise need to be hired (e.g. computer scientist, software engineer, graphics designer)
Define scope	Establish the budget for development, the necessary equipment, the required licenses, the personnel, etc.
Feedback system	Create a system of rewards and penalties for the decisions made by the player. Consider whether points, objects, feedback, among others, will be used. Establish an algorithm that marks the objectives and learning outcomes within the game. Either by a linear or branched algorithm. Define minimum elements for the achievement of the objectives.
Verify functionality	Use each of the components of the game and make sure it works as expected.
Evaluation	Evaluate with an instrument that measures usage satisfaction, gameplay, learning perception, and design. Assess whether the target population acquired the knowledge and skills intended to be achieved

5. **Iterate & Refine**:
    - Modify the game based on feedback.
    - Repeat testing and refining as necessary.

4.10.2 Best-Practice Production and Application:

- **Balanced Challenge**: The game should be challenging but not so difficult that it frustrates learners.
- **Immediate Feedback**: Offer real-time feedback on in-game decisions to reinforce learning.

- **Relevance**: Ensure the game's scenarios and challenges are authentic and relevant to real-world medical practice.
- **Integration**: Tie the game to other instructional methods, using it to complement lectures, readings, or simulations.
- **Continuous Update**: Medicine evolves. Ensure that the game content remains current and accurate.

4.10.3 Relevant Pedagogical Theories [22]

- **Constructivism**: Games often involve active problem-solving, allowing learners to construct knowledge through in-game actions and decisions.
- **Motivation Theory**: Games incorporate elements like scores, badges, and leaderboards that can boost learner motivation [47].
- **Experiential Learning**: **Kolb's** experiential learning theory emphasises learning through action and reflection, both integral in GBL.

See Chap. 1 for detailed descriptions of these relevant learning theories.

In conclusion, game-based learning in HPE has the potential to enhance learner engagement, motivation, and retention. The effectiveness of GBL, grounded in several pedagogical theories, makes it a valuable approach, especially for topics that benefit from active problem-solving and repeated practice. Proper design, integration with other learning methods, and ongoing updates are crucial for its success.

4.11 Social Media in HPE

The use of platforms such as YouTube [48], TikTok [49], and Instagram [50, 51] for HPE is a relatively new phenomenon, but its rapid rise in popularity, especially among younger generations, has prompted educators to explore its potential. While extensive research specifically on TikTok in HPE might be limited due to its novelty, there are emerging studies and anecdotes. For example, as of August 2, 2020, the hashtag "MedEd" has over 4.6 million views on TikTok [49]. Content ranges from discussing anatomy lessons to breaking down concepts learned in medical school, Objective Structured Clinical Examination (OSCE) stations or clinical skills and demonstrating lifesaving procedures [49]. These platforms provide a sense of community by allowing users to respond to videos and follow others with similar interests. YouTube, TikTok and Instagram have 'reels' which allow for shorter, high-yield content with a focus on rapid identification of key points and engaging presentations. General limitations of using social media to spread medical information have been discussed previously and include issues with undisclosed conflicts of interest, unchecked spread of misinformation, difficulty identifying source credibility, and the need to filter through large amounts of noise and false information. Another challenge is that some platforms like TikTok restrict videos to 60 seconds or less, limiting the depth of information conveyed in a given video [52]. Moreover, unfamiliarity with the platform and time and research required to design and create videos that consider the components of efficacious multimedia design impact the practicality and feasibility of implementation.

4.11.1 Practical Step-by-Step Instructions for TikTok Creation

1. **Identify Objectives**:
   - Decide on the educational message or skill you wish to convey (Table 4.5).
2. **Plan Content**:
   - Due to TikTok's time constraint (typically 15–60 s), content should be concise and focused.
3. **Recording**:
   - Use a good quality smartphone or camera.
   - Ensure proper lighting.
   - Consider using tripods or stabilisers for steady shots.
4. **Editing**:
   - Use TikTok's built-in editing tools or external apps to trim and add captions, effects, or music. Canva also has a variety of templates.
5. **Engagement**:
   - Utilise trending hashtags relevant to the content.
   - Collaborate with popular medical educators or influencers for wider reach.

Table 4.5 Design principles for creating TikTok videos (adapted from Lacey [52])

Consideration	Description
Catchy title	Clear title outlining topic and learning outcomes
Concise material	Concise coverage of core concepts and learning outcomes, aligned with curricula
Relevant material	Avoid redundant material and assumption of prior knowledge
Conversational tone	Relaxed pacing and tone. Narrative storytelling, spoken in human voice.
Thematic consistency	Consistent design principles and templates, including colour, music, layout and font
Appropriate visuals	Maximise use of graphics and images and highlight important content with arrows and colour. Instructor images avoided.
Frequency of releases	Regular and consistent publishing schedule and frequent publishing of content
Feedback	Gain student feedback and modify future designs and content accordingly
Follow up material	Captions with links to further content, resources, including self-assessment

6. **Publish & Monitor**:
   - Regularly check comments and engage with viewers.
   - Address queries or misconceptions that may arise.

4.11.2 Best-Practice Production and Application

- **Ethical Considerations**: Ensure patient confidentiality and privacy. Never share identifiable patient information.
- **Accuracy & Credibility**: As with any educational resource, content should be evidence-based and accurate. Avoid spreading misinformation.
- **Engagement**: Use engaging visuals, demonstrations, or storytelling techniques to capture viewers' attention (Fig. 4.6).
- **Continuous Learning**: Stay updated with TikTok trends and incorporate them when relevant to increase engagement.
- **Feedback Loop**: Encourage feedback from peers and learners to refine and improve content over time.

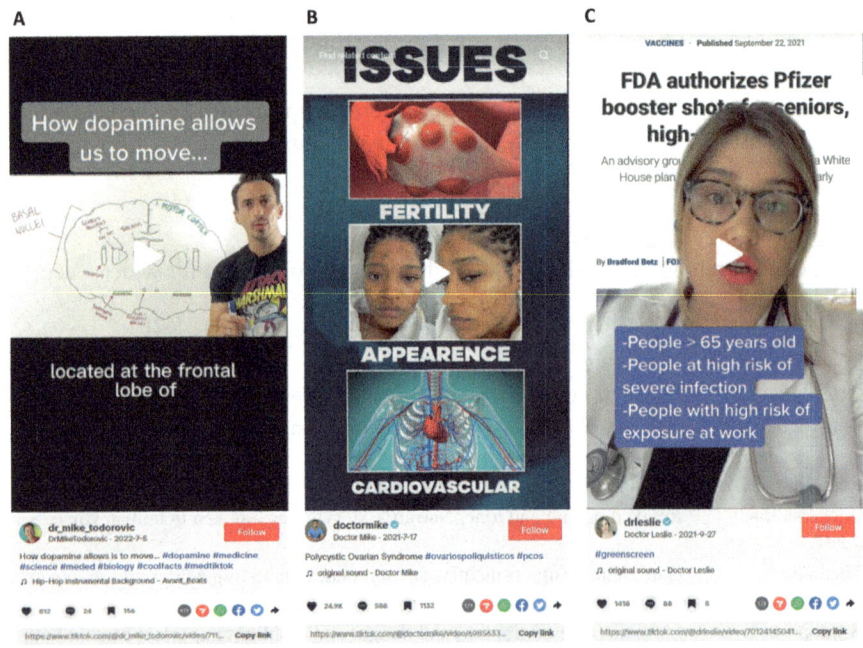

Fig. 4.6 Medical influencers on TikTok for the #MedEd hashtag. (**a**) Dr Todorovic explaining the role of a hormone using whiteboard illustration. (**b**) Dr Mike discussing the polycystic ovarian syndrome symptoms. (**c**) Dr Leslie discussing the criteria for the COVID-19 booster vaccination

4.11.3 *Relevant Pedagogical Theories*

- **Social Learning Theory**: Learners often observe and emulate behaviours or techniques showcased by others, and TikTok, with its short video format, is a platform ripe for such observational learning [22].
- **Cognitive theory of multimedia learning**: Simultaneous presentation of visual and audio features and highlighting content with arrows, graphics and colours create high-yield outcome-focussed content, avoiding extraneous material and promoting student engagement. When using narrative, a relaxed tone spoken in a human voice, avoiding instructor images increases accessibility and relatability of material and avoids unnecessary intrinsic load [7–9].
- **Microlearning**: Platforms like TikTok and Instagram with short videos fit the microlearning trend, where content is delivered in small, focused segments [49].
- **Communities of practice**: Virtual communities allow for users to develop, retrieve, and explore content generated by others at their convenience, irrespective of time or place. Social media enhances relationships, allowing people to share, discuss, and debate a wide variety of interests and key issues with colleagues and experts from around the world [53].

See Chap. 1 for detailed descriptions of these relevant learning theories.

Case Study
During the COVID-19 pandemic, the use of TikTok by medical professionals to disseminate facts and dispel myths related to the disease was a huge topic of discussion. Many users developed content to clarify questions about the disease. These videos have reached millions of viewers and gained popularity, most notably a video receiving more than one million views on how to properly don and doff gloves. In another example, medical professional, Dr. Rose Marie Leslie (@drleslie), has used TikTok to share videos on topics such as the symptoms of COVID-19, which has been viewed 4.3 million times [49] (Fig. 4.6c).

In conclusion, social media platforms like the TikTok format provide an avenue for quick, engaging bursts of HPE. Its potential is significant, especially in reaching younger audiences or those outside traditional HPE pathways. As with any tool, it is essential to use it responsibly, ensuring the content is both educational and ethically produced. As TikTok's use in HPE is still emerging, continuous evaluation and adaptation are crucial.

4.12 Tips and Tricks

- **Student engagement**—use a variety of technologies to create engaging, interactive, and immersive learning experiences that enhance student motivation and participation.

- **Appropriateness**—when deciding on which learning tool to use, it is crucial to consider which tool is most appropriate for the type of teaching material.
- **Pedagogical alignment**—consider the underlying pedagogy and use evidence-based approaches when designing educational material around a specific tool, ensuring that it aligns with the educational goals and curriculum objectives.
- **Adequate resourcing**—identify whether you have the appropriate budget, equipment, technology, expertise and/or collaborators to accomplish the desired goal. Consider the cost implications and strive for solutions that provide a good return on investment without compromising educational quality.
- **Security and privacy**—ensure that any technology used complies with legal and ethical standards for data security and privacy, particularly when handling sensitive student information.
- **Upfront evaluation**—develop evaluation methods and identify key measure and metrics to collect, during the design phase.
- **Feedback and assessment**—provide real-time feedback and incorporate robust assessment tools to evaluate student progress and learning outcomes.
- **Pilot testing**—be prepared to pilot test projects with a small sample of the target audience, as well as colleagues who may adopt the tool.
- **Faculty training**—provide adequate training and support for educators to effectively integrate and utilize the technology in their teaching.
- **Continuous quality improvement**—continue to iterate and quality improve tools based on the feedback received and evaluation results.
- **Accessibility and inclusivity**—ensure the technology is accessible to all students, including those with disabilities or limited access to high-end devices and internet connections.
- **Dissemination plan**—have a dissemination plan in place for the sharing of learnings and results from the implementation—this may be institutional presentations, abstracts, conferences and publications.
- **Recognition and ongoing support**—seek recognition for innovations through award and grant applications.
- **Pedagogical relevance and best practice**—often, educators put their desire to lead innovation with a specific tool above the best practice application. It is important to consider whether the tool is appropriate for the task and enhances value (engagement versus distraction).
- **Technology overuse**—sometimes there can be an overreliance on technology which can undermine fundamental skills and critical thinking if not balanced well. Technology use should also not come at the expense of necessary human interaction between students and with educators.
- **Constructive alignment**—the application of the tools should be mapped and aligned to the desired learning outcomes, so that students understand why and how the tool should be used. Consider how to standardise assessment around the innovation as well.
- **Costs involved**—consider the initial investment of purchasing new technology, developing digital content, and maintaining any infrastructure. Also account

upfront for ongoing costs for regular updates, technical support, subscriptions etc.
- **Time commitment**—developing innovative education with new tools can be time consuming. Ensure you have support, approval and awareness from your supervisors of the time investment required. Have a plan in place for covering existing workloads.
- **Educator training and support**—educators may need training and ongoing professional development and support to integrate the technologies into their teaching.
- **Technical issues**—products need to be regularly checked for glitches, software and hardware issues, and ensure that capacity for integration, scalability, and compatibility is maintained, as technology advances.
- **Quality improvement**—tools need to be constantly quality improved and adapted to changing trends, curriculum revisions, software updates, and tested for bug fixes.
- **Access and equity**—note that not all students will have equal access to technologies or high-speed internet. When designing, consideration must be given to accessibility requirements for inclusivity.
- **User resistance**—be aware of resistance to change in both educators and students due to comfort, familiarity, time and effort required for the learning curve and fear of the unknown.
- **Ethics, privacy and security**—when collecting personal information from users, ensure that you have the appropriate approvals, security measures, and compliance with legal and regulatory requirements.
- **Evaluation of outcomes**—educators often forget to design the evaluation before the implementation of the tool, which is essential to test utility and effectiveness of the tool.
- **Knowledge translation**—Educators fall short on sharing learnings and tips with the broader educational community through knowledge translation and dissemination

4.13 Conclusion

Selecting the appropriate digital tool for various educational contexts is a nuanced and critical decision. It requires a thorough understanding of the specific learning objectives, the target audience, and the benefits and limitations of the pedagogical approach. The choice of technology should align with the desired outcomes, enhancing the learning experience and promoting engagement. In some cases, simulation and virtual reality may be ideal for hands-on skill development, while other scenarios might benefit from the interactivity of gamification or the flexibility of podcasts. The integration of artificial intelligence, such as chatbots, can provide personalised support, while social learning tools can encourage collaboration and knowledge sharing. The key is to consider the unique needs of the educational setting and the preferences of both educators and learners. As technology continues to evolve, staying informed about emerging tools and evidence-based practices is essential to make informed decisions about the right digital tools for the job. Ultimately, the thoughtful selection of digital tools can significantly enhance the educational experience and better prepare learners for the challenges they will face in their respective fields.

References

1. Ahmet A, et al. Is video-based education an effective method in surgical education? A systematic review. J Surg Educ. 2018;75(5):1150–8.
2. Hurtubise L, et al. To play or not to play: leveraging video in medical education. J Grad Med Educ. 2013;5(1):13–8.
3. Harrington CM, et al. 360° operative videos: a randomised cross-over study evaluating attentiveness and information retention. J Surg Educ. 2018;75(4):993–1000.
4. Dong C, Goh PS. Twelve tips for the effective use of videos in medical education. Med Teach. 2015;37(2):140–5.
5. Krumm IR, et al. Making effective educational videos for clinical teaching. Chest. 2022;161(3):764–72.
6. Bada D, Olusegun S. Constructivism learning theory: a paradigm for teaching and learning. J Res Method Educ. 2015;5(6):66–70.
7. Mayer RE. Incorporating motivation into multimedia learning. Learn Instr. 2014;29:171–3.
8. Moreno R, Mayer RE. Cognitive principles of multimedia learning: The role of modality and contiguity. J Educ Psychol. 1999;91(2):358–68.
9. Mayer RE, Moreno R. Nine ways to reduce cognitive load in multimedia learning. Educ Psychol. 2003;38(1):43–52.
10. McSparron JI, Vanka A, Smith CC. Cognitive learning theory for clinical teaching. Clin Teach. 2019;16(2):96–100.
11. Young JQ, et al. Cognitive load theory: implications for medical education: AMEE Guide No. 86. Med Teach. 2014;36(5):371–84.
12. Mayer RE. Cognitive theory of multimedia learning. In: The Cambridge handbook of multimedia learning. 2nd ed. New York: Cambridge University Press; 2014. p. 43–71.
13. Yue C, et al. Applying the cognitive theory of multimedia learning: an analysis of medical animations. Med Educ. 2013;47(4):375–87.
14. Mayer RE. Using multimedia for e-learning. J Comput Assist Learn. 2017;33(5):403–23.
15. Cuevas J, Dawson BL. A test of two alternative cognitive processing models: learning styles and dual coding. Theory Res Educ. 2017;16(1):40–64.
16. Issa N, et al. Applying multimedia design principles enhances learning in medical education. Med Educ. 2011;45(8):818–26.
17. Lai-Kwon J, et al. Designing a wholly online, multidisciplinary Master of Cancer Sciences degree. BMC Med Educ. 2023;23(1):544.
18. Kok DL, et al. Screen-based digital learning methods in radiation oncology and medical education. Tech Innov Patient Support Radiat Oncol. 2022;24:86–93.
19. Latif MZ, et al. Use of smart phones and social media in medical education: trends, advantages, challenges and barriers. Acta Inform Med. 2019;27(2):133–8.
20. Mukhalalati B, et al. Applications of social theories of learning in health professions education programs: a scoping review. Front Med. 2022:9.

21. Boulos MNK, Maramba I, Wheeler S. Wikis, blogs and podcasts: a new generation of Web-based tools for virtual collaborative clinical practice and education. BMC Med Educ. 2006;6(1):41.
22. Taylor DCM, Hamdy H. Adult learning theories: implications for learning and teaching in medical education: AMEE Guide No. 83. Med Teach. 2013;35(11):e1561–72.
23. Goldie JG. Connectivism: a knowledge learning theory for the digital age? Med Teach. 2016;38(10):1064–9.
24. Hodson N. Landscapes of practice in medical education. Med Educ. 2020;54(6):504–9.
25. Tang KS, et al. Augmented reality in medical education: a systematic review. Can Med Educ J. 2020;11(1):e81–96.
26. Sutherland J, et al. Applying modern virtual and augmented reality technologies to medical images and models. J Digit Imaging. 2019;32(1):38–53.
27. Yeung AWK, et al. Virtual and augmented reality applications in medicine: analysis of the scientific literature. J Med Internet Res. 2021;23(2):e25499.
28. Bin S, Masood S, Jung Y. Chapter twenty - virtual and augmented reality in medicine. In: Feng DD, editor. Biomedical information technology. 2nd ed. Academic Press; 2020. p. 673–86.
29. Vaughan N, et al. A review of virtual reality based training simulators for orthopaedic surgery. Med Eng Phys. 2016;38(2):59–71.
30. Moro C, et al. The effectiveness of virtual and augmented reality in health sciences and medical anatomy. Anat Sci Educ. 2017;10(6):549–59.
31. Dhar P, et al. Augmented reality in medical education: students' experiences and learning outcomes. Med Educ Online. 2021;26(1):1953953.
32. Kok DL, et al. Virtual reality and augmented reality in radiation oncology education - a review and expert commentary. Tech Innov Patient Support Radiat Oncol. 2022;24:25–31.
33. Lopreiato JO, Sawyer T. Simulation-based medical education in pediatrics. Acad Pediatr. 2015;15(2):134–42.
34. Battista A, Nestel D. Simulation in medical education: evidence, theory, and practice. 2018;151–162.
35. Simulation in medical education: brief history and methodology Principles and Practice of Clinical Research, 2015;1(2).
36. Horcik Z. Renewing the tools for simulation-based training in medical education: how situated approaches can help us? 2022. p. 61–80.
37. Rencic J, et al. A situated cognition model for clinical reasoning performance assessment: a narrative review. Diagnosis. 2020;7(3):227–40.
38. Mitchell SA, Boyer TJ. Deliberate Practice in Medical Simulation, in StatPearls. StatPearls Publishing; 2024. Copyright © 2024, StatPearls Publishing LLC.: Treasure Island (FL) ineligible companies. Disclosure: Tanna Boyer declares no relevant financial relationships with ineligible companies.
39. Ericsson KA. Deliberate practice and the acquisition and maintenance of expert performance in medicine and related domains. Acad Med. 2004;79(10 Suppl):S70–81.
40. Berk J, et al. Medical education podcasts: where we are and questions unanswered. J Gen Intern Med. 2020;35(7):2176–8.
41. Newman J, et al. Podcasts for the delivery of medical education and remote learning. J Med Internet Res. 2021;23(8):e29168.
42. Lomayesva NL, et al. Five medical education podcasts you need to know. Yale J Biol Med. 2020;93(3):461–6.
43. Kaplan H, Verma D, Sargsyan Z. What traditional lectures can learn from podcasts. J Grad Med Educ. 2020;12(3):250–3.
44. Argueta-Muñoz FD, et al. Instructional design and its usability for branching model as an educational strategy. Cureus. 2023;15(5):e39182.
45. McCoy L, Lewis JH, Dalton D. Gamification and multimedia for medical education: a landscape review. J Am Osteopath Assoc. 2016;116(1):22–34.

46. Krishnamurthy K, et al. Benefits of gamification in medical education. Clin Anat. 2022;35(6):795–807.
47. Kapp K. The gamification of learning and instruction: game-based methods and strategies for training and education. San Francisco, CA: Pfeiffer; 2012.
48. Curran V, et al. YouTube as an educational resource in medical education: a scoping review. Med Sci Educ. 2020;30(4):1775–82.
49. Comp G, Dyer S, Gottlieb M. Is TikTok the next social media frontier for medicine? AEM Educ Train. 2021;5(3)
50. Essig J, et al. InstaHisto: utilizing instagram as a medium for disseminating visual educational resources. Med Sci Educ. 2020;30(3):1035–42.
51. Koenig JFL, et al. Using Instagram to enhance a hematology and oncology teaching module during the COVID-19 pandemic: cross-sectional study. JMIR Med Educ. 2021;7(4):e30607.
52. Lacey H, Price JM. #MedEd-The 'TikTok' frontier of medical education. Clin Teach. 2023;20(5):e13636.
53. Yarris LM, et al. Finding your people in the digital age: virtual communities of practice to promote education scholarship. J Grad Med Educ. 2019;11(1):1–5.

Chapter 5
Teaching and Facilitating Online

Alicia Mew, Bhaumik Shah, and David L. Kok

Abstract Teaching in the online space is a unique and challenging experience but can also be incredibly rewarding. In this chapter, we dive into the various aspects of online teaching, from design to direct instruction and facilitation. We will provide theoretical models and practical advice for a beginner online educator, with a particular focus on how application of a Community of Inquiry model and the principles of Transformative Learning can enhance online teaching. We will highlight the multiplicity of roles included in the identity of an online teacher and suggest various ways to acquire skills and competencies to perform them effectively, thus providing the building blocks for educators to adapt as facilitators of online learning and cultivate an environment that ignites transformative growth and change in learners.

Key Points
- Educators are the catalysts for change, responsible for shaping future healthcare leaders by challenging them to exceed current norms and improve patient care.
- The Community of Inquiry model provides a sound theoretical framework for organising and evaluating online teaching.
- Different roles, identities and skills are needed to teach in the online space.
- Teacher presence and effective facilitation are crucial to the success of online education.

A. Mew
Victorian Comprehensive Cancer Centre, Melbourne, VIC, Australia

B. Shah
University of Melbourne, Melbourne, VIC, Australia

Epworth Hospital, Melbourne, VIC, Australia

D. L. Kok (✉)
University of Melbourne, Melbourne, VIC, Australia

Peter MacCallum Cancer Centre, Melbourne, VIC, Australia

Monash University, Melbourne, VIC, Australia
e-mail: dkok@unimelb.edu.au

© The Author(s), under exclusive license to Springer Nature Switzerland AG 2025
D. L. Kok et al. (eds.), *Best Practices in Online Education*, IAMSE Manuals, https://doi.org/10.1007/978-3-031-90349-6_5

5.1 Introduction

Teaching in the online space is a unique and challenging experience but can also be incredibly rewarding. Being an effective online educator is not just about having knowledge and skills; it's also about embracing being a teacher as an identity and understanding your role and responsibilities to create a learner-centred online education experience. It is now widely accepted that effective education requires more than simply transferring knowledge from teacher to student—the accumulation of facts and figures is not enough to make a lasting impact on behaviour change in practice. Thus, for teachers to make a meaningful impact on learners, we need to adopt progressive teaching methodologies that inspire learners to undergo significant personal and intellectual growth.

In this chapter, we'll dive into the various aspects of online teaching, from design to direct instruction and facilitation. We will provide theoretical models and practical advice for a beginner online educator with a particular focus on how the application of a Community of Inquiry model and the principles of Transformative Learning can enhance online teaching. We will highlight the multiplicity of roles included in the identity of an online teacher and suggest various ways to acquire skills and competencies to perform them effectively.

5.2 Embracing a Teacher's Identity

Educators hold a privileged and unique role in society, and this is especially true in health professional education (HPE). Educators are the catalysts for change and make an appreciable impact on healthcare outcomes by educating future health professionals and challenging them to move beyond the norms and conventions that are currently in place to continuously improve and innovate in patient care. As advocates of change, an educator's mission is to pass on our refined skills, research, and knowledge and hence to raise up others while also helping them to avoid the pitfalls and challenges that are only obvious through experience. We aspire to spark motivation and inspire passion in learners that can then translate into excellence in their daily practice. However, if we are to truly be these catalysts of change, we must first foster change within ourselves and embrace the identity of an online teacher.

Change, much like effective teaching, is a layered process that starts small and builds momentum over time (as seen in Fig. 5.1: Depth of Change). It begins at the individual level, where personal awareness, skills, and mindsets are developed. As individuals embrace change, it expands to groups—teams, committees, or classrooms—where collective actions and shared goals can lead to significant impact. Finally, the ripple effect of change reaches the organisational level, where systemic transformations take hold, influencing policies, practices, and culture. Educators play a vital role in facilitating this progression, inspiring learners to not only adopt change individually but also to collaborate and innovate within their teams and, ultimately, their professional communities.

Fig. 5.1 Depth of Change

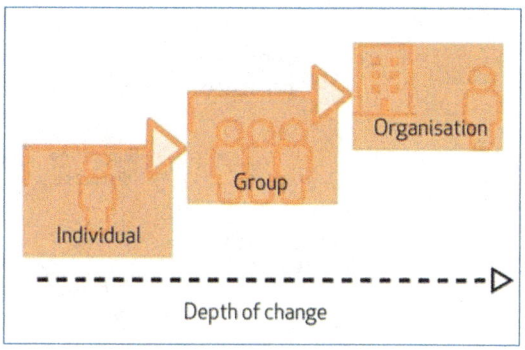

Effective teaching remains the cornerstone of successful online learning, yet it is often underestimated. The role of an online teacher can be challenging as it no longer conforms to the expectations of teachers that have been established for millennia. The 'sage on the stage' is replaced by a multitude of learning items and activities, of which the teacher is just one. This has implications on many levels, including the students' perception of the teacher, the teacher's perception of themselves and the 'presence' which the teacher has in the classroom. Understanding and embracing that this presence is different to that from traditional teaching is the first step an online educator must take. Understanding the components of this presence is also important to be able to enhance it. The Community of Inquiry framework is one way in which this can be understood.

5.3 Community of Inquiry Framework

"The Community of Inquiry framework is a collaborative-constructivist process model that describes the essential elements of a successful online higher education learning experience." (Castellanos-Reyes, 2020, p. 1) [1]

The Community of Inquiry (COI) framework was developed in the late 1990s by Randy Garrison, Terry Anderson, and Walter Archer at the University of Alberta, Canada. Recognising the rise of digital learning, they aimed to enhance communication between teachers and learners. [1] The COI framework consists of three essential elements, termed presences: cognitive presence, social presence, and teaching presence (See Fig. 5.2). These elements collaboratively foster engagement and motivation in online courses and the coordination of all three is critical for successful online learning. [1, 2] We focus here on the teaching presence which plays a pivotal role in orchestrating the three elements. The teaching presence encompasses the educator's active involvement in facilitating learning, guiding discussions, providing feedback, and establishing a supportive online learning environment. This active presence of the teacher is integral to creating meaningful interactions, promoting deep learning, and ultimately driving positive change in learners' understanding and perspectives. [2]

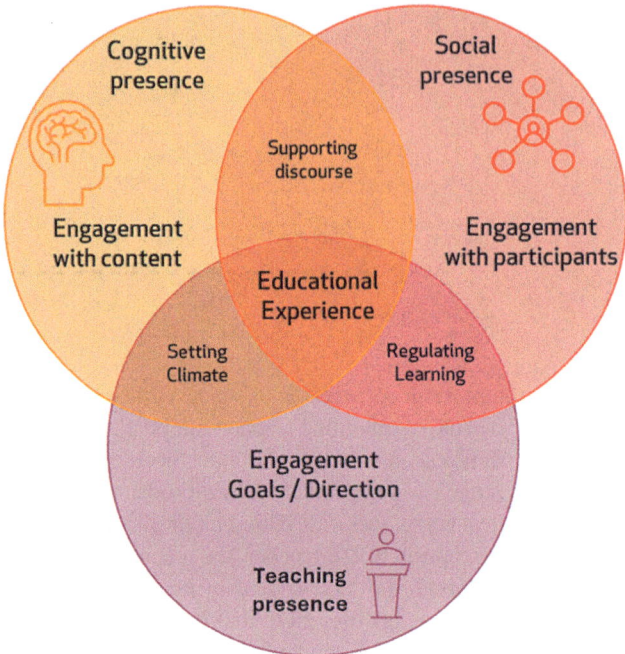

Fig. 5.2 The Community of Inquiry Framework

The COI framework closely aligns with Mezirow's concept of transformative learning (introduced in Chapter 1 and further described below), particularly in how it defines the role of teaching presence. The teaching presence in the COI framework embodies this transformative role. Teachers do not merely convey information but actively facilitate meaningful interactions and reflective processes that drive learners towards transformative insights and changes in perspective. [3]

5.3.1 Teaching Presence: The Roles and Responsibilities of the Online Educator

Online educators need to perform a multiplicity of roles, and this is particularly important within the COI framework as the teaching presence encompasses the design, facilitation, and guidance of cognitive and social processes to achieve meaningful educational outcomes [4]. The teaching presence starts before the course begins with learning design and can continue throughout the course through facilitation, mentoring and direct instruction. [4]

5 Teaching and Facilitating Online

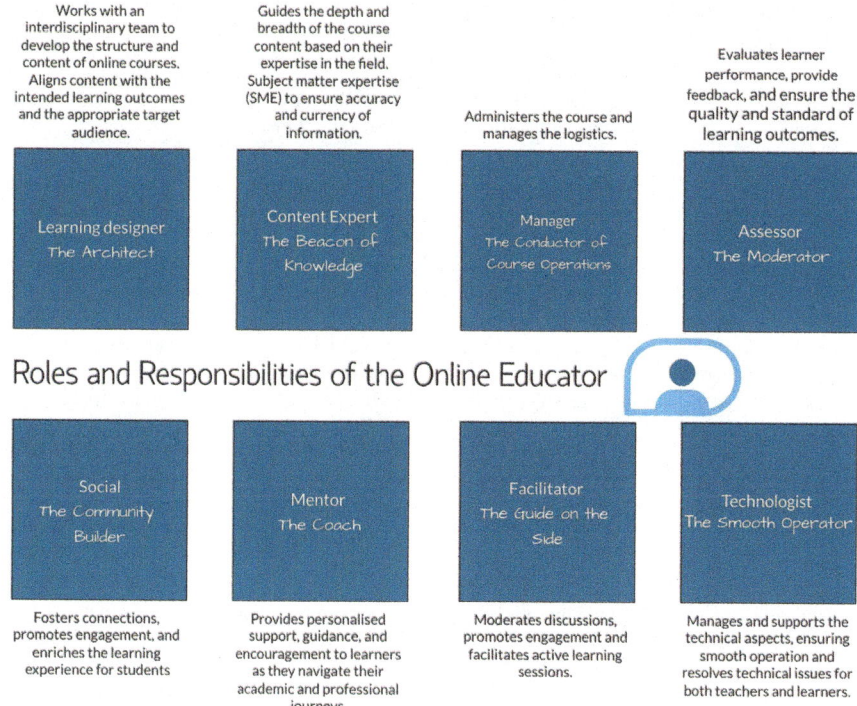

Fig. 5.3 Roles and Responsibilities of the Online Educator

In the context of health professional education, these roles have been described in diverse ways. Figure 5.3 outlines the roles that one may need to encompass to provide a comprehensive online learning experience that is structured and provides relevant learning experiences. Depending on institutional and course-related contexts, you might need to undertake some or all of these roles. Additionally, there might be a hierarchical structure within the faculty, determining which roles you need to assume, especially in co-teaching scenarios [3–8].

5.3.2 Tasks of the Online Educator

These roles, responsibilities and tasks align with the COI framework's emphasis on teaching presence, which includes design and organisation, facilitation and direct instruction (Table 5.1).

Table 5.1 Roles and Common Tasks of the Online Educator

Learning designer Architect of Educational Experience	Content Expert The Beacon of Knowledge	Manager The Conductor of Course Operations	Assessor The Moderator
• Collaborate with subject matter experts to pinpoint essential topics and gather current, pertinent educational resources such as articles, videos, simulations, and case studies. • Structure content sequentially to support a coherent learning journey. • Apply instructional design strategies to foster captivating and dynamic learning modules. • Ensures content inclusivity, accessibility, and alignment with educational goals. • Present course materials in various accessible formats, adhering to universal design principles. • Develop a detailed grading rubric that clearly defines criteria for each grade level, ensuring transparency and fairness. • Clearly convey course objectives, protocols, and optimal practices to educators.	• Highlight key emerging trends and research findings succinctly. • Clearly define essential topics, learning objectives, and assessments for subject mastery. • Develop concise course content, including lectures, readings, and case studies. • Design assessments that directly align with learning objectives. • Conduct thorough reviews to maintain course material quality and relevance. • Lead focused workshops or training sessions to efficiently share expertise.	• Updates timetables, due dates, and assessment expectations. • Provide tips and support tailored to individual learner needs and learning styles. • Ensure prompt email responses and implement a systematic approach to managing late submissions and inactivity. • Coordinate class management effectively for both synchronous and asynchronous sessions, utilising digital tools for efficiency. • Manages faculty leaves and turnover. • Utilise feedback, evaluation, and data analysis to assess and enhance the effectiveness of online courses. • Continuously improve courses based on learner feedback, research findings, and the integration of emerging technologies.	• Apply grading criteria, rubrics, and standards to assess the quality and accuracy of learners' work. • Provide timely grading of assignments. • Participate in regular calibration meetings to discuss and align grading standards among educators. • Set specific time frames for grading and feedback to manage workload and ensure prompt communication. • Direct learners to additional resources, tutorials, and guides that can be accessed to improve their understanding of the subject matter.

(continued)

Table 5.1 (continued)

Learning designer Architect of Educational Experience	Content Expert The Beacon of Knowledge	Manager The Conductor of Course Operations	Assessor The Moderator
Social The Community Builder	Mentor The Coach	Facilitator The Guide on the Side	Technologist The Smooth Operator
• Build rapport and connection with teachers, peers and the learning environment. • Utilise icebreakers and introductions to foster a welcoming, inclusive atmosphere. • Engage students through storytelling, humour, and anecdotes to spark interest and curiosity. • Keep ongoing, active communication. • Provide timely, individualised support to create a nurturing learning environment. • Promote collaborative learning and problem-solving with group activities and projects. • Give constructive feedback and guidance for both academic and personal growth. • Demonstrate effective communication skills, including active listening, empathy, and clear expression.	• Personalised one-on-one guidance. • Pastoral care provision. • Navigation support for online resources and networks. • Academic, career, and personal development assistance. • Constructive feedback on learner progress and work. • Expertise sharing in relevant subject areas.	• Craft and facilitate engaging discussion prompts. • Moderate online discussions to align with educational goals. • Employ interactive techniques to boost student participation. • Foster critical thinking and reflection in learners. • Establish clear netiquette guidelines. • expectations. • Utilise diverse teaching strategies for varied learning preferences. • Maintain consistent online engagement and support for learners. • Guide students through course material and complex ideas.	• User-friendly learning platform, accessible to all. • Guide on ed-tech and LMS for content delivery, interaction, and assessment. • Manage and support the technical aspects of the online learning platform. • Assure operational smoothness and technical issue resolution. • Assist with navigation of the online learning platform and integrated technology effectively. • Continuous updates on educational technology trends.

5.4 Adult Transformative Learning

Jack Mezirow formulated the transformative learning theory in the late 1900s. This theory explains how individuals engage in critical self-reflection to evaluate their beliefs and experiences, ultimately evolving from limited perspectives. Mezirow's focus lies in understanding individuals' worldviews and the catalysts driving shifts in their perceptions of the world [9, 10].

Transformative learning theory is based on andragogy principles. It has two primary assumptions: learners are adults, and are capable of rational thought and discourse [10–12]

Like Knowles (14), the father of andragogy, Mezirow (10) and Cranton (13) acknowledge that adults possess a set of experiences, beliefs, and assumptions that influence their perception of the world. Adults actively shape their learning experiences, they can choose and define their expectations, perceptions, thoughts, and emotions and are self-directed learners driven by their own needs and interests. Adults bring their existing beliefs and experiences into the learning process, which serves as a foundation for new learning, however, this can also lead to the rejection of new ideas that do not conform to their preconceptions. Transformative learning principles emphasise the importance of challenging these preconceptions and embracing a more inclusive and reflective approach. Adults thrive in an environment that is supportive, collaborative, and respectful of their autonomy but must be challenged with practical application and real-world problem-solving to allow them to integrate new experiences and perspectives into their understanding, fostering personal growth and development [10, 12–15].

5.4.1 Transformative Change

Mezirow identifies ten phases that constitute the process of transformative learning which provides a structured approach to understanding how learners can achieve profound shifts in perspective [16]:

Mezirow's Transformative Learning Theory provides a framework for developing a mindset conducive to change, allowing individuals to embrace new learning experiences and adapt to evolving circumstances. Mezirow's 10 phases of transformative learning (1978) have been compiled into a seven-phase in Fig. 5.4, which provides an insight of how adults learn and can change their perspectives [15, 17].

One of the biggest examples of transformative learning in education faculty development is the COVID-19 pandemic when educators globally were presented with a "disorienting dilemma". The pandemic caused a rapid shift in the delivery of education and created a crisis moment that highlighted the inadequacies of traditional teaching methods in the new context of online learning. The "disorienting dilemma" prompted many to question the relevance and effectiveness of their current pedagogical approaches, and they began experimenting with various online

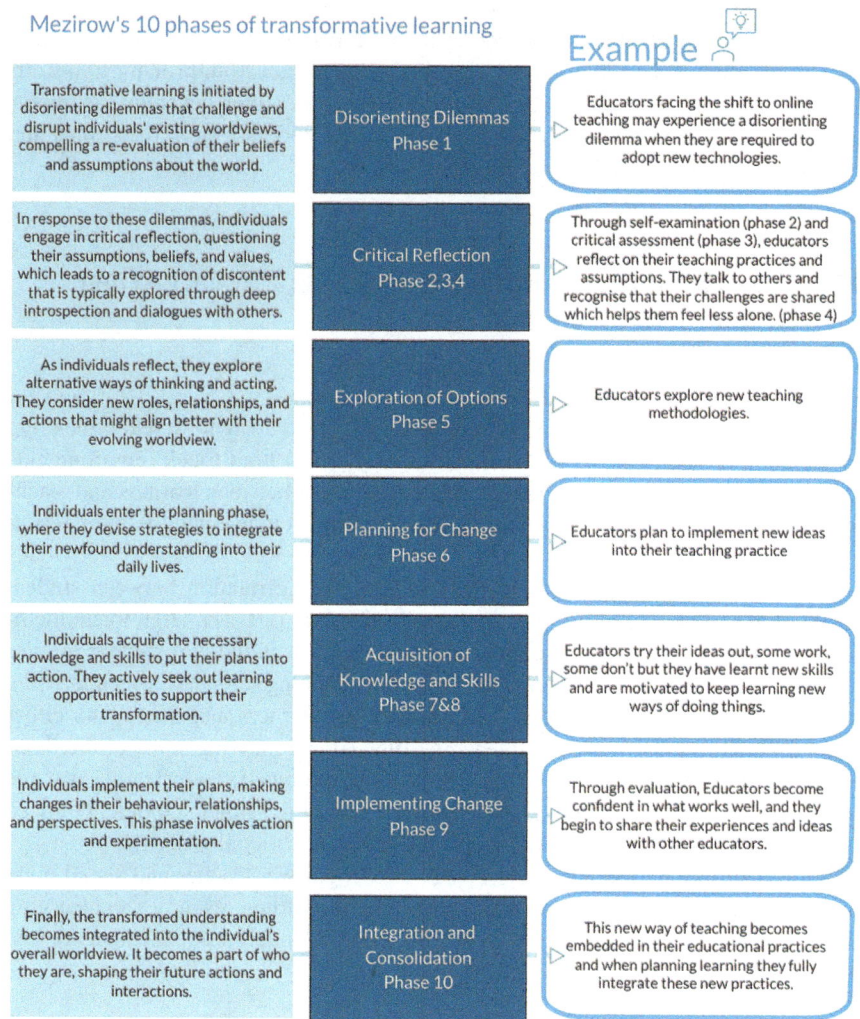

Fig. 5.4 Mezirow's 10 phases of transformative learning linked to Andragogy [11, 15, 16]

tools and platforms to facilitate remote learning. Experts in online learning were called in to provide professional development, communities of practice consisting of interprofessional teams were established and there was a period of trial-and-error where different methods were tested to see what worked best for their learners. The transition required educators to undergo transformative learning, which involved a fundamental shift in their thinking, feelings, and actions about what it means to be an educator in today's digital age. Educators quickly become proficient with educational technologies and learning management systems (LMS). Tools like Zoom, Google Classroom, and Microsoft Teams became essential for delivering content and maintaining communication with learners and courses were restructured to include more interactive elements. This transformative change led to several positive outcomes, mainly that the support systems, skills and knowledge of delivering education online were adopted into all facets of education from primary to university teaching strategies and practices. Educators became acutely aware of the importance of maintaining a strong teacher presence and understanding their roles and responsibilities in the online learning environment. [11, 18, 19]

5.5 Thoughtful Incorporation of Teaching Presence When Online Designing Curricula

Like all aspects of an online HPE curriculum, there is no single set formula for optimal online teaching, and we have deliberately stayed away from recommending a specific approach. Online instruction can vary from 'high touch' environments where there is a substantial interaction and engagement between learners and teachers to 'low touch' where there is minimal (or no) direct engagement between teachers and learners.

The research data suggests that there is a strong correlation between student satisfaction and increased teaching and social presence [20, 21]. High touch methods also provide more opportunities for responding to individual student queries and thus offering tailored learning experiences. That being said, high-touch learning is not without its downsides—interaction between learners and instructors either requires synchronously scheduled teaching time (thus removing some of the flexibility of online educational techniques) or, if asynchronous, exposes learners to time delays in correspondence and therefore runs the risk of missing the moment of need when the learners' brain is actively engaged in the educational process.

Thus, deciding on the appropriate degree of cognitive, teacher and social presence will be highly individualised depending on your setting, resources and learning objectives. Some considerations that can be used to guide these decisions are discussed in the following section:

5.5.1 Factors Influencing Teaching Approach

Online education might look quite different based on the students, teachers, and subject related factors. Some of the variables are described in Table 5.2. They can provide unique affordances or challenges.

Table 5.2 Important Factors to Define Context of Online Education

Factor	Scenario	Impact
Delivery mode	Completely online	Allows more affordance for working students and global audiences.
	Mixed	Social presence is improved with some face-to-face sessions. Teachers get better nontextual cues.
Student cohort background	Homogenous	Does not need a differentiated teaching approach. Less concern about equity.
	Interprofessional	Can lead to more diverse discussions and more nuanced point of view.
Competing roles	Full time student	Less stressors for work/life/study balance
	Working students	More insight from work experience. More pastoral care (counselling) needed.
Mode of activities	Fully asynchronous	More flexibility for students.
	Includes synchronous activities (e.g. webinars)	Less efforts needed to maintain social presence.
Duration of the study	Short courses (3 months or less)	A bird's eye view of other subjects and overall plan of course would be needed. Handover and networking with other subject coordinators needed.
	Long courses	You get to know students better during longer courses. Formative assignments are feasible for longer courses.
Geography	Local cohort	No concerns about time zone considerations for synchronous contents and deadlines.
	Global cohort	The content and assignments need to be tailored for the whole cohort. More diverse discussions with comparison and contrasting possible.
Teaching staff	Single person	No need for consensus meetings for grading. No regular catch ups needed to stay on same page.
	Team	Depending on hierarchy in teaching faculty they might assume distinct roles. Subject coordinator might take more managerial, mentor and subject expert role. A tutor might take a more facilitator role. More diversity of ideas. More confidence in failing a student. Debriefing, skill building and coaching for fresh staff is feasible.
Experience with the subject	Teachers new to the subject	Takes time to familiarise with content, activities and common pitfalls.
	Teacher with prior experience with the subject	Can be more efficient in managerial and research roles (subject renewal, content/assignment/rubric changes).

5.5.2 Examples

A 2-hour online short course is designed to upskill ward staff in ultrasound techniques to assist with difficult intravenous cannulations. Its expected audience is clinical staff with busy ward jobs engaging in self-directed professional development in their own time. The course materials are otherwise fully asynchronous with a mix of videos, text and simple on-screen interactives. It is foreseen to be a high-volume, rapid-throughput course. Given that the learner cohort is likely to be at highly variable times, the level of learning complexity is not high, the design team opts for a low-touch (less interactive) design, with only a limited asynchronous discussion board feature.

A 3-year online Master's degree for Health Professionals aims to upskill its participants in all areas with cardiac health. There is a suite of core and elective subjects covering a range of highly complex and detailed learning materials. Intake levels are expected in the range of 30–40 students per subject operating within normal university semester time periods. Given the relatively regulated teaching hours, complexity of material and higher level of resourcing, a high-touch teacher presence (more interactive) design is adopted, with weekly webinars, discussion boards, direct student email contact and video logs (Vlogs).

5.6 Continuous Maintenance of Competencies as an Online Educator

The role of an online educator can often feel more isolating compared to traditional face-to-face teaching. A considerable proportion of new online educators may not have prior experience in online learning environments as a student and thus frequently acquire their skills through on-the-job experiences. However, numerous opportunities exist to develop the requisite knowledge and skills for effective online teaching supported by transformative learning principles. According to Mezirow's transformative learning theory, critical reflection, discourse, and action are essential for profound changes in professional practice. [15, 17] Institutions and educators themselves can facilitate these opportunities through structured support, peer collaboration, and self-directed learning.

5.6.1 Communities of Practice and Transformative Peer Learning

Collaboration with colleagues is one of the rich sources of professional development for online educators. Mezirow emphasises the role of critical reflection, discourse, and action in transformative learning. [17] As educators transition from

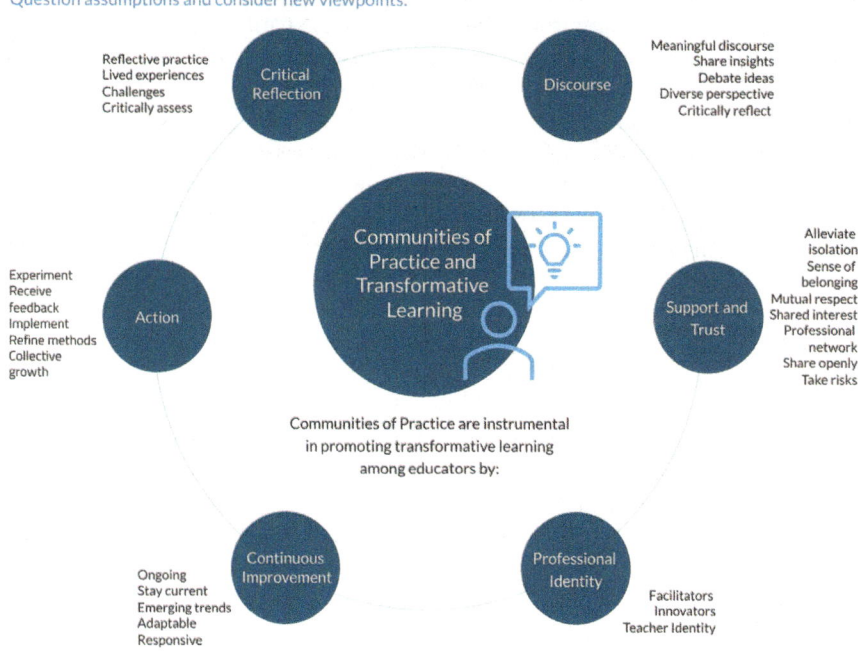

Fig. 5.5 Communities of Practice and Transformative Learning

traditional to online education, they face challenges that necessitate questioning and reshaping their understanding of instructional design. Communities of Practice (CoP) act as valuable support networks where educators can share experiences, concerns, and expertise, prompting collaborative learning and trust. This allows educators to reflect on their experiences, challenge assumptions, and experiment with new instructional strategies. This process fosters a transformative shift in their professional identity and teaching methods. Building CoPs is crucial for professional growth, especially in the rapidly evolving landscape of online education, where educators must continuously adapt to meet the needs of online learners. CoPs enable educators to stay current with educational trends and technologies and develop new skills, enhancing both individual and collective teaching practices [18, 22, 23] (Fig. 5.5).

5.6.2 Co-Teaching

Online courses involving co-teaching provide a fertile ground for mutual learning and professional growth. Like CoPs, co-teaching offers opportunities for transformative elements by allowing educators to share experiences, reflect on their practices, and learn from each other. However, this is only possible if all educators involved are willing to learn from each other, establish parity, and address interpersonal dynamics [24]. Regularly scheduled consensus meetings for assignments and planning synchronous and asynchronous activities are key collaborative practices. These meetings facilitate the exchange of insights and suggestions for improving course content and delivery. Systematic debriefing sessions after each teaching activity provide a platform for critical reflection, where co-teachers can discuss what worked well or not and why. This reflective practice is central to Mezirow's theory, promoting continuous improvement and adaptation.

5.6.3 Self-Directed Learning

Online educators can also engage in self-directed learning by exploring resources such as academic journals, online courses, and professional development webinars. This proactive approach enables educators to continuously reflect on and refine their teaching strategies, staying current with the latest trends and technologies in online education.

5.7 Institutional Support for Online Educators

Institutions, depending on their budget and the breadth of their online course offerings, can play a pivotal role in supporting the professional development of online educators by providing training programs, workshops, and resources that assist educators in critically reflecting on their existing practices and adapting to new teaching modalities.

Table 5.3 highlights some key mechanisms to support online educators:

5.8 Tips and Tricks

- **Be familiar with the content, assessments, technical requirements, and IT support resources**. Facilitate transformative learning effectively by connecting content to learners' experiences and perspectives. [6]
- **Regularly update a profile of your student cohort** to understand their backgrounds, needs, and potential barriers (e.g., cultural and linguistic diversity (CALD), age, (dis)ability, technology issues, geographic/time zone issues).
- **Maintain regular and consistent teaching presence which includes:**
  - Being approachable and accessible through synchronous "office hours" and other means.

Table 5.3 Key mechanisms to support online educators

Tools for Teaching Alleviate the workload of online educators by providing effective tools to enhance and support online teaching so that educators can focus more on teaching and learning engagement.	• User-friendly platforms such as a high-quality LMS that facilitate streamlined and seamless communication channels with learners. • Automated grading systems and feedback systems aligned with grading rubrics. • Learning analytics: An effective LMS also enables the tracking of learner engagement aiding in the early identification of disengaged or at-risk students. • Institutional subscriptions to software for synchronous webinars, reference management, and assignment preparation (e.g. virtual presentations) and feedback
Mentoring and Peer Support: Foster a sense of community among online educators by encouraging collaboration, knowledge sharing and networking.	• Establish mentorship programs where experienced online educators guide newer faculty members. • Establish Communities of Practice (CoP) to provide peer support networks.
Technical Support: Streamline processes and reduce manual workload and technical challenges by providing robust technical support to allow for better design and implementation of both synchronous and asynchronous teaching activities.	• Provide technical support for online platforms, tools, and software including help desk and IT specialist. • Provide 24/7 tech support to remove barriers for an international cohort of students. • Live technical support during synchronous webinars and assistance with organising active learning sessions are critical for both the learning experience and the teacher.
Quality Assurance Maintain efficiency, reliability, and precision in online learning delivery to ensure a consistent learning experience across courses.	• Develop clear guidelines for course design, assessment, and evaluation. • Regular reviews of online courses ensure alignment with learning objectives and quality standards. • Set clear expectations regarding the expected time commitment for various activities and optimal turnaround times for feedback delivery
Formal Education: Empower educators with the necessary knowledge and skills to excel in online teaching.	• Create online resource centres with curated materials, templates, and guides for designing and delivering online courses. For example: comprehensive staff guides or manuals that introduce faculty to the features of the LMS, commonly used resources, typical activities, and troubleshooting procedures. • Offer ongoing professional development opportunities for online educators. For example: workshops, guest lectures, and the dissemination of scholarly articles.

This table has been adapted from [25–28]

- Focusing on pastoral care and supporting students' emotional needs for learning and, in particular, disengaged "silent learners". Regular synchronous engagements can provide insights into well-being through non-verbal cues.
- Facilitation, not just instruction, guide discussions. Ask probing questions to help students critically reflect and transform their perspectives.

- Encouraging peer learning and interaction to build a supportive community where students feel safe to share, challenge their views and gain multiple perspectives.
- Maintain regular asynchronous communication via emails and announcements. Templates can streamline this process (e.g., no submission, plagiarism/AI input flagged, inactivity).
- Adapt content and teaching based on student feedback, ensuring that the content remains relevant and engaging and shows teacher responsiveness.

- **Familiarise yourself with LMS features**. Use learning analytics to track student engagement and identify issues early (e.g., time spent in learning environment, delayed submissions, inactivity) and contact students proactively.
- **Promote active learning** through digital tools like breakout rooms and interactive platforms to help learners articulate their thoughts, confront their beliefs, and consider alternative viewpoints.
  Educate students about academic integrity and the consequences of plagiarism and inappropriate AI use. Incorporate collaborative projects where accountability is shared, and team members are encouraged to support one another in upholding ethical practices, such as proper citation and equal contribution.
- **Design assessments that require critical analysis and personal reflection**, making them less amenable to AI-generated responses. Model transparency when using AI-generated templates for planned announcements.
- **Keep notes and provide handovers** on what worked and what did not for new coordinators to ensure continuity, address any concerns, maintain a stable learning environment, and smooth transitions to the next iterations of the subject.
- **Build a community of educators** for regularly sharing advice, debriefing, and innovating. This collaborative approach enhances the collective ability to facilitate transformative learning. It can also provide much needed support as online educators can be at greater risk of burnout.

5.9 Conclusion

In conclusion, the evolving landscape of online education presents both unique challenges and profound opportunities for educators. As education transitions from traditional teaching methods to transformative approaches within online environments, our role as educators must evolve to embracing a learner-centred philosophy. The integration of the Community of Inquiry (CoI) framework and Mezirow's Transformative Learning Theory is critical for creating effective online education environments that promote deep learning and personal growth. Both frameworks emphasise essential aspects of teaching and learning that, when combined, can significantly enhance the quality of online education by providing the structural elements necessary for creating a supportive learning environment and the processes needed to facilitate personal change in learners. This integration fosters a supportive community that encourages collaboration, reduces isolation, and enhances the overall learning experience.

By combining these theories, educators can ensure that online is not merely about content delivery but also about facilitating meaningful learning experiences that lead to lasting change, improving educational outcomes and better preparing learners for their future careers and roles in our ever-changing society. Effective online teaching requires a multifaceted approach, incorporating multiple roles that educators should play. Institutional support, including access to professional development, technical assistance, and collaborative communities of practice, is crucial for sustaining the growth and effectiveness of online educators. These support systems enable educators to continuously refine their skills and adapt to the ever-changing demands of the digital learning landscape.

It is essential to realise that your own teaching context can influence the practical accommodations that you need to make for effective online education.

Ultimately, embracing the identity of a teacher as a catalyst for change is essential. By fostering a culture of transformative learning, we not only enhance the educational experience for our learners but also contribute to the development of future leaders capable of making a meaningful impact in their respective fields. Through dedication, innovation, and a commitment to continuous improvement, educators can navigate the complexities of online teaching and inspire transformative growth in their learners.

References

1. Castellanos-Reyes D. 20 Years of the community of inquiry framework. TechTrends Link Res Pract Improve Learn. 2020;64(4):557–60.
2. Rosser-Majors ML, Rebeor S, McMahon C, Wilson A, Stubbs SL, Harper Y, et al. Improving retention factors and student success online utilizing the community of inquiry framework's instructor presence model. Online Learn J. 2022;26(2):6.
3. Garrison DR, Anderson T, Archer W. Critical inquiry in a text-based environment: computer conferencing in higher education. Internet High Educ. 1999;2(2–3):87–105.
4. Anderson T, Rourke L, Garrison R, Archer W. Assessing teaching presence in a computer conferencing context. Online Learn [Internet]. 2019 [cited 2024 May 28];5(2). Available from: https://olj.onlinelearningconsortium.org/index.php/olj/article/view/1875
5. EdD BB. Eight roles of an effective online teacher [Internet]. Faculty Focus | Higher Ed Teaching & Learning. 2013 [cited 2024 May 29]. Available from: https://www.facultyfocus.com/articles/online-education/online-course-delivery-and-instruction/eight-roles-of-an-effective-online-teacher/
6. Conklin S, Dikkers AG. Instructor social presence and connectedness in a quick shift from face-to-face to online instruction. Online Learn. 2021;25(1):135–50.
7. Salmon G. E-tivities: the key to active online learning. Routledge; 2013.
8. jessica.critten. University of Colorado. 2021 [cited 2024 May 29]. Strategies for Promoting Teaching Presence in your Online Courses. Available from: https://www.cu.edu/blog/online-teaching-blog/strategies-promoting-teaching-presence-your-online-courses
9. Christie M, Carey M, Robertson A, Grainger P. Putting transformative learning theory into practice. Aust J Adult Learn. 2015;55(1):9–30.

10. Mezirow J. Transformative learning. New Dir Adult Contin Educ. 1997;74(74):5–12.
11. Rojo J, Ramjan L, George A, Hunt L, Heaton L, Kaur A, et al. Applying Mezirow's transformative learning theory into nursing and health professional education programs: a scoping review. Teach Learn Nurs. 2023;18(1):63–71.
12. Stansberry SL. A systematic mapping of literature on transformative learning theory in educational technology. In: Spector JM, Lockee BB, Childress MD, editors. Learning, design, and technology [Internet]. Cham: Springer International Publishing; 2023. p. 1459–78. [cited 2024 May 20]. Available from: https://link.springer.com/10.1007/978-3-319-17461-7_159.
13. Cranton P. Understanding and promoting transformative learning: s guide to theory and practice. Routledge; 2016.
14. Knowles MS. The modern practice of adult education; Andragogy versus Pedagogy. 1970.
15. Kitchenham A. The evolution of John Mezirow's transformative learning theory. J Transform Educ. 2008;6(2):104–23.
16. Mezirow J. Learning to think like an adult. Learn Transform Crit Perspect Theory Prog. 2000:3–33.
17. Mezirow J. How critical reflection triggers transformative learning. Adult Contin Educ Teach Learn Res. 2003;4:199.
18. Brennan A, Gorman A. Leading transformative professional learning for inclusion across the teacher education continuum: lessons from online and on-site learning communities. Prof Dev Educ. 2023;49(6):1117–30.
19. O'Dea X (Christine), Stern J. Virtually the same?: Online higher education in the post COVID-19 era. Br J Educ Technol. 2022;53(3):437–442.
20. Martin F, Bolliger DU. Engagement matters: student perceptions on the importance of engagement strategies in the online learning environment. Online Learn [Internet]. 2018 Mar 1 [cited 2024 Sep 18];22(1). Available from: https://olj.onlinelearningconsortium.org/index.php/olj/article/view/1092
21. Gay GH, Betts K. From discussion forums to eMeetings: integrating high touch strategies to increase student engagement, Academic Performance, and Retention in Large Online Courses. Online Learn [Internet]. 2020 Mar 1 [cited 2024 Sept 18];24(1). Available from: https://olj.onlinelearningconsortium.org/index.php/olj/article/view/1984
22. Ahmed N, Tabb A. An analysis of the role of communities of practice in transformational learning during a pandemic. In: 45th Annual Conference Proceedings. ERIC; 2021. p. 6.
23. Wenger E. Communities of practice: learning, meaning, and identity [Internet]. 1st ed. Cambridge University Press; 1998 [cited 2024 Jun 4]. Available from: https://www.cambridge.org/core/product/identifier/9780511803932/type/book
24. Kim E, Pratt SM. Co-teaching goes online: the impact of virtual co-teaching on the practices of a co-teaching partnership during COVID. Stud Teach Educ. 2024;20(1):107–27.
25. Rotar O. Online student support: a framework for embedding support interventions into the online learning cycle. Res Pract Technol Enhanc Learn. 2022;17(1):2.
26. Stone C. Improving student engagement, retention and success in online learning. In: Shah M, Kift S, Thomas L, editors. Student retention and success in higher education: institutional change for the 21st century [Internet]. Cham: Springer International Publishing; 2021. p. 167–89. Available from:. https://doi.org/10.1007/978-3-030-80045-1_9.
27. Picciano A. Theories and frameworks for online education: seeking an integrated model. Online Learn. 2017:21.
28. Roddy C, Amiet DL, Chung J, Holt C, Shaw L, McKenzie S, et al. Applying best practice online learning, teaching, and support to intensive online environments: an integrative review. Front Educ. 2017;2:59.
29. Boettcher JV, Conrad RM. The online teaching survival guide: simple and practical pedagogical tips. John Wiley & Sons; 2021.
30. Boettcher JV. Ten core principles for designing effective learning environments: Insights from brain research and pedagogical theory. Innov J Online Educ [Internet]. 2007 [cited 2024 Jun 7];3(3). Available from: https://www.learntechlib.org/p/171446/

31. Zhang J, Chen H, Wang X, Huang X, Xie D. Application of flipped classroom teaching method based on ADDIE concept in clinical teaching for neurology residents. BMC Med Educ. 2024;24(1):366.
32. Kim S, Choi S, Seo M, Kim DR, Lee K. Designing a clinical ethics education program for nurses based on the ADDIE model. Res Theory Nurs Pract. 2020;34(3):205–22.
33. Khoshnoodifar M, Zangiabadian M, Ilaghi M. Design, implementation and evaluation of a systematic review course for medical students. Strides Dev Med Educ. 2023;20(1):129–34.
34. Salmon G, Tombs M, Surman K. Teaching medical students about attention deficit hyperactivity disorder (ADHD): the design and development of an E-learning resource. Adv Med Educ Pract. 2019:987–97.
35. Sait S, Tombs M. Teaching medical students how to interpret chest x-rays: the design and development of an e-learning resource. Adv Med Educ Pract. 2021:123–32.
36. Overbaugh RC. based guidelines for computer-based instruction development. J Res Comput Educ. 1994;27(1):29–47.
37. Branch R. Common instructional design procedures organized by ADDIE. In: Instructional design: the ADDIE approach [Internet]. 1st ed. Boston: Springer; 2009. p. 1–5. Available from:. https://doi.org/10.1007/978-0-387-09506-6_1.
38. De Lima DPR, Gerosa MA, Conte TU, de M. Netto JF. What to expect, and how to improve online discussion forums: the instructors' perspective. J Internet Serv Appl. 2019;10(1):22.
39. Al-Fraihat D, Joy M, Masa'deh R, Sinclair J. Evaluating E-learning systems success: an empirical study: Comput Hum Behav. 2019;102.

Chapter 6
Multidisciplinary, Interdisciplinary and Interprofessional Online Education

David Seignior, Michelle Barrett, and David L. Kok

Abstract Interprofessional Collaborative Practice (IPCP) in which multiple health professionals from diverse professions work together to improve patient care, is increasingly common clinical practice. Therefore, interprofessional education (IPE) is an ever more important part of health professional education (HPE). Online interprofessional education (OIPE) provides logistical and pedagogical benefits (and challenges) for diverse HPE cohorts, learning not just in parallel, but with, from and about each other. This chapter differentiates between multidisciplinary, interdisciplinary and interprofessional education, and while focusing on the latter, is relevant to all.

This chapter outlines key theories underpinning effective OIPE such as the Contact hypothesis, and the Community of Inquiry model, and how these can help in the design and delivery of effective and 'safe' learning experiences for interprofessional cohorts. The chapter consider various IPE curriculum frameworks and essential IPCP skills, knowledge and capabilities, but also how to support learners' 'dual identity' development as inter(professional) practitioners.

The importance of teaching presence, and the skills, knowledge and support required to design and facilitate interprofessional learning through synchronous and asynchronous engagements are highlighted. The chapter concludes with a focus on online learning activities specifically relevant to enhancing and assessing IPCP, such as virtual multidisciplinary team meetings (MDTM), interprofessional case discussions, reflective and interprofessional group assessment tasks.

D. Seignior (✉)
University of Melbourne, Melbourne, Australia
e-mail: david.seignior@unimelb.edu.au

M. Barrett
Victorian Comprehensive Cancer Centre, Melbourne, Australia

D. L. Kok
University of Melbourne, Melbourne, Australia

Peter MacCallum Cancer Centre, Melbourne, Australia

Monash University, Melbourne, Australia

© The Author(s), under exclusive license to Springer Nature Switzerland AG 2025
D. L. Kok et al. (eds.), *Best Practices in Online Education*, IAMSE Manuals, https://doi.org/10.1007/978-3-031-90349-6_6

Key Points
- Online Interprofessional education (OIPE) has the same challenges and benefits as regular online HPE, but also more of both.
- The aim of OIPE is to enhance Interprofessional collaborative practice (IPCP) i.e. learning with, from, and about other professions (multidisciplinary education is learning with other professions in parallel).
- Contact hypothesis [1], is a key theory underpinning IPE, whereby (intergroup) interprofessional relationships can be enhanced by 'contact' with other professions, under certain conditions.
- The Community of Inquiry model [2] and, cognitive, social and teaching presences are important to consider for OIPE design and delivery.
- There are three main types of IPE, formal, informal and serendipitous. This chapter focuses on formal (intentional) IPE.
- OIPE can be delivered in wholly online, blended, or hybrid formats and can be anything from a 2-hr program to part of a 2-year master's degree, pre, or post-licensure and with varying combinations of professions.
- Various frameworks guide IPE/OIPE curriculum, which generally include understanding and working respectively with one's own and other professions to advance patient care, communication and relationship building and team dynamics.
- Teaching presence, including design, direct instruction, facilitation [3] and 'therapeutic presence' [4] are vital elements of OIPE.
- Teaching OIPE requires a complex array of knowledge and skills integrating interprofessional education and online learning. This is often enhanced through team-teaching.
- OIPE benefits from a combination of both asynchronous and synchronous engagements, i.e. self-directed learning and discussions and real time webinars.
- Assessments which consider the process not just the result of interprofessional collaboration, including reflective and group tasks, are greatly beneficial in OIPE.

6.1 Introduction

Previously, we have focused on designing and teaching online HPE more generally. In this chapter, we home in on the design and delivery of online HPE for learners from diverse disciplinary and/or professional backgrounds, and in particular, online interprofessional education (OIPE). We begin by briefly addressing why OIPE is an increasingly important aspect of HPE and defining key terms before exploring some of the basic pedagogical theories and frameworks that underpin it. We then look at key considerations and fundamentals for designing and teaching IPE, such as program type (wholly online, blended or hybrid) and duration; teacher's knowledge, skills, and support; learner level, experience, and profession; and relevant curriculum, pedagogy (including assessment) and technology. Concepts will be demonstrated in application through case studies taken from real-life.

IPE requires understanding, support and resourcing at all levels, from higher policy and professional organisations to teaching institutions, including faculty, discipline, course/subject and teachers and students. Here, we assume that the necessary systemic and organisational approvals are in place and that this is aimed at those at the faculty level either planning a new OIPE program, adjusting or putting an existing in-person IPE, partly or wholly online. However, we also hope it presents a compelling case for policy and decision-makers, on the benefits of OIPE.

6.1.1 Interprofessional Collaborative Practice

The aim of OIPE is to enhance Interprofessional collaborative practice (IPCP). IPCP has become more important in clinical contexts, given an increase in chronic illnesses such as cancer and overburdened and under-resourced healthcare systems. IPCP is intended to achieve the 'quadruple aim' of optimising patient safety, experience, and clinical outcomes, as well as HP wellbeing and cost-efficiency [5].

The WHO defines IPCP as:

> When multiple health workers from different professional backgrounds provide comprehensive services by working with patients, their families, carers and communities to deliver the highest quality of care across settings [6].

To achieve better IPCP, it makes sense that HPs spend at least part of their education and training, learning together with other professions or disciplines. This is now common in most nursing and allied health education and is also becoming increasingly integrated into medical education, which has traditionally taken a more unidisciplinary approach. Given the logistical complexities of bringing together learners from different courses, faculties, campuses and even institutions, online interprofessional education (OIPE) has become an increasingly popular way of delivering this type of learning. Beyond the logistical and economical advantages, other advantages of OIPE, as well as its specific challenges, are discussed below.

6.1.2 Definitions

The term *interprofessional* is often used interchangeably with *multidisciplinary*, *interdisciplinary*, and *transdisciplinary*, and while there are some commonalities, their differences have pedagogical, not just semantic implications, and it is important to understand their differences when designing and delivering OIPE.

We do not differentiate between *discipline* and *profession* here when it comes to designing and teaching education for diverse HPE cohorts, i.e. we will consider inter*professional* and inter*disciplinary* education as one and the same. However, it is important to distinguish between the prefixes *inter* and *multi* as, in this context,

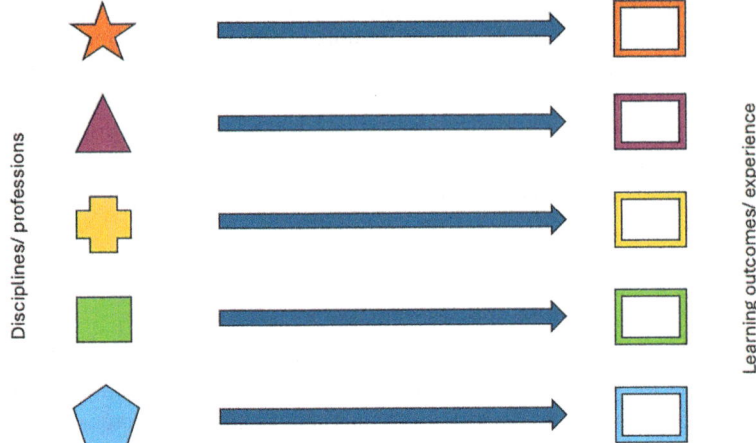

Fig. 6.1 Multidisciplinary or multiprofessional education

they refer to very different types of learning interaction that will influence program design and delivery.

The essential difference between *multi*disciplinary and *inter*disciplinary (or *multi*professional and *inter*professional) is the degree to which interaction and integration between disciplines (or professions) occurs. In *multi*disciplinary or *multi*professional education, learners from different disciplines or professions learn together 'in parallel' without necessarily interacting (See Fig. 6.1), with each other. So, learning from, with and about learners from other disciplines or professions are not intended learning outcomes.

*Inter*disciplinary or *inter*professional education on the other hand, requires interaction with students from other disciplines or professions, learning about their diverse range of skills, knowledges, and perspectives i.e., collaborating, with the aim of integrating this approach into clinical contexts (See Fig. 6.2).

As defined by the Center for the Advancement of Interprofessional Education (CAIPE):

> Interprofessional education occurs when two or more professionals learn with, from and about each other to improve collaboration and the quality of care [7].

6.1.3 Why OIPE?

Given it is a more complex endeavour, we focus here on designing and teaching online *interprofessional* education (OIPE), although most concepts will also apply to multidisciplinary contexts. As well as the pros and cons of online HPE covered in earlier chapters, there are additional benefits and challenges that apply specifically to OIPE, and we will touch upon these now.

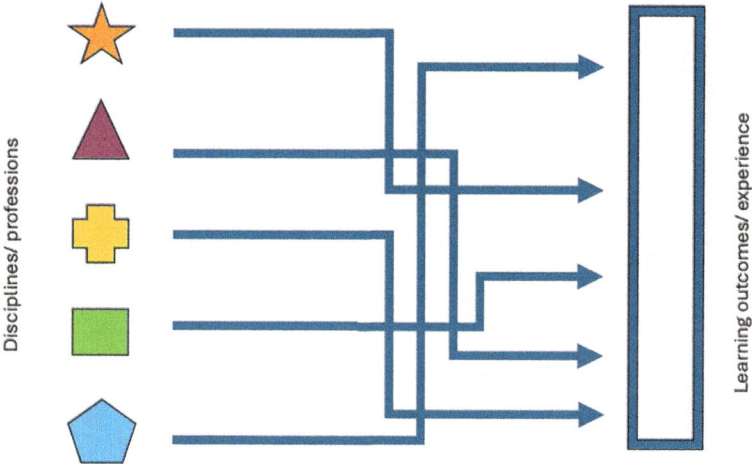

Fig. 6.2 Interdisciplinary or interprofessional education

Overcoming Logistical and Economical Challenges

The likelihood of a geographically and temporally dispersed cohort is greater when students are coming from different professions, faculties, campuses and even institutions. Similarly, coordinating timetables for multiple and 'crowded' discipline curricula can be especially difficult with IPE. The flexibility and convenience of OIPE are especially advantageous in overcoming these logistical obstacles, for students, teachers, and institutions. However, as noted above, the advantages of OIPE go beyond the logistical and economical.

Levelling the Playing Field

A key theory underpinning IPE is referred to as the Contact hypothesis [1], which suggests that 'intergroup relations' can be improved, and 'intergroup conflict' can be reduced through 'contact' with 'outgroups' (e.g., other professions) under certain conditions. These include, among other things, equal status, collaboration towards a 'superordinate goal' and institutional support, all of which can be facilitated to some degree by an online environment.

While health professions are always evolving, their organisational structures and cultures are often largely hierarchical, with asymmetrical power relationships existing in the interactions between many of the disciplines. This can affect workplace dynamics and increase risks of miscommunication, anxiety, feelings of 'imposter syndrome' and 'silencing' of certain professions. It can also result in tension and even conflict, all of which can negatively affect HP workers and, ultimately patient welfare. There is evidence to suggest that the nature of online engagement, particularly through asynchronous modes such as discussion threads (but also in synchronous webinars), can minimise professional (and other) status differences, reduce anxiety, and allow for more inclusive, non-hierarchical interprofessional interactions [8]. This is due in part to the lack of embodied signifiers of status that exist with in-person interactions, but also the 'psychological distance and safety' and

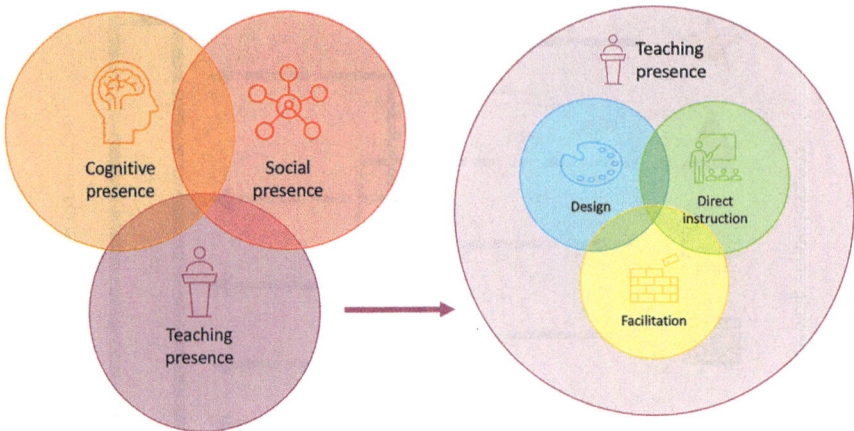

Fig. 6.3 Community of Inquiry

time for reflection and considered responses that asynchronous online presence allows. This can help learners to understand how professions, including their own, fit into an interprofessional collaborative context and, therefore, develop confidence and agency that transfers to the in-person clinical environment. Thus, OIPE can play an important role in improving interprofessional dynamics in the clinical workplace.

6.1.4 Interprofessional Communities of Inquiry

The opportunities for 'safe' contact with learners from other professions, using a social constructivist approach [9] is a key aspect of IPE, as learning to 'work with' other professions and understand their roles, responsibilities, and priorities, are as important as specific skills such as communication, and leadership. The Community of Inquiry Framework [2] discussed in Chap. 1 is particularly helpful for an interprofessional cohort. While the 'three presences', cognitive, teaching and social, as shown in Fig. 6.3, must all be considered, teaching and social presence are of particular importance for interprofessional cohorts.

OPIE requires learning activities (including assessments), that enable meaningful social and cognitive presence, guided by authentic and consistent teaching presence. OIPE can provide both the necessary interactions with other professions and the time for self-paced learning, considered communication, reflection, and dual-identity development (as both professional and interprofessional practitioners) needed for effective IPCP [10].

OIPE Collaborative Learning Tools
In Chap. 4, we explored various digital learning tools and techniques which apply equally to OIPE. However, there are some tools especially useful for OIPE, including interactive IP simulations, videos and role plays, and live interactions such as

webinar-based multidisciplinary team meetings (MDTs). These also model online clinical practices such as telehealth, virtual MDTs, etc., which are increasingly popular post-COVID. OIPE means learners can access the learning from any location, including their workplace, which is convenient and enables opportunities for workplace integrated learning.

A final benefit of online IPE, also not often considered, is the access to 'student analytics' now built into all learning management systems (LMS). While detailed data on how students are engaging with learning content and each other is beneficial for designing any course of learning, it can be particularly so for IPE. This is because of the ability to map peer-to-peer interactions using tools and theories such as Actor Network Theory (ANT) [11], which provide data on the nature of interprofessional interactions that can inform teaching and design.

6.1.5 Types of IPE

Having established its importance, we now turn to what OIPE looks like. There are generally considered to be three broad types of IPE: formal, informal, and serendipitous [12].

- **Formal IPE** is undertaken within a formal HP education or training program, where interprofessional learning outcomes are intended, stated, and prioritised. For example, a specific IPE subject or training module within an allied health or medical course.
- **Informal IPE** is usually within an education or training program, but where interprofessional learning is not necessarily intended or stated as the main learning outcome. For example, a subject within a course where the cohort is from diverse HPs but where the focus is on another topic, e.g., cancer sciences, and any IPE is incidental.
- **Serendipitous IPE** is any ad hoc interprofessional learning that occurs within a clinical context or an HP education or training program. For example, an unexpected educational encounter in a multidisciplinary team meeting, where something is learnt with, from and/or about another professional.

6.1.6 Wholly Online or Blended OIPE

The next consideration is about whether the IPE program is to be wholly online or blended, i.e., a combination of online and in-person learning or hybrid (face-to-face with simultaneous synchronous online webinar). In essence, IPE has a role to play in any context and learning environment in which HPE is being delivered.

The specific benefit and best application depend on the context of the IPE and considerations such as:

- Is it IPE for a particular clinical scenario, such as surgery or intensive-care, or a more general context?
- Is it focusing on a particular aspect of IPE, such as team dynamics during patient rehabilitation or patient discharge medication communication?
- Is it introducing IPE to learners with limited or no in situ clinical experience or experienced clinicians?
- Are the learners working in the clinical environment at the same time?
- What type and quality of online technology is available?

While it may be preferable, and in some cases necessary for IPE to take place in person, if not in situ (real-world healthcare settings), most interprofessional interactions can be learnt and practiced online, as the COVID-19 pandemic has taught us. Even interprofessional aspects of 'hands-on' clinical scenarios, such as surgery, can be learnt online, for example, 'understanding roles, responsibilities and priorities of surgical teams', or participating in interprofessional pre-operative planning. As VR and AR technologies become more widely accessible, 'hands-on' activities will be increasingly simulated and taught online [13].

Which approach taken will largely be decided by practical, logistical factors such as the geographical locations and preferences of the learners (and teachers), their availability, the duration of the program and the context of the learning. In some ways, it is helpful to see all IPE as blended and on a spectrum rather than a binary because even a wholly online IPE program will need workplace integration, where learners apply what they learn in a clinical context. Conversely, in-person IPE will undoubtedly have some online elements.) Again, we focus here on wholly online IPE, as it can be readily adapted to a blended approach and should always consider integration into the in-person clinical, patient-care context.

6.2 Which Professions Should Do OIPE?

There is limited literature on which professions (and how many, in which combinations) should undertake IPE, let alone IPCP. Increasingly non-healthcare professionals such as information technologists and medical technicians are now involved in IP teams. Patients (consumers) and even family and carers are now also being considered as potential members of IP teams and, therefore, as teachers and students of IPE.

The professional constitution of an IPE cohort is largely dependent on the IPCP context it is preparing learners for and, therefore, the specific intended learning outcomes as well as the experience and capabilities of the teacher. If the IPE is for a particular context or aspect of IPCP, then it makes sense that it is limited to relevant professions. On the other hand, for general IPE learning, one could argue for a 'more the merrier' approach, as one can never learn too much or about too many professions.

When deciding on the professional make-up of the learner cohort, consider the professional background and experience of the teachers. While it is not essential (or possible) for teachers to be familiar with the perspectives of all HPs in their cohort, it is necessary for them to at least be confident that they can accommodate a profession's perspective and facilitate their relevant involvement in that specific learning context. This is discussed in detail below.

6.2.1 Pre or Post Licensure?

Is IPE more effective and beneficial for undergraduate/ prelicensure or postgraduate/post licensure learners? On this, the academic jury is out, but it is fair to say there are pros and cons to each. The main argument either way centres on identity formation and the aim to help a learner develop a "dual identity" [10] as both a professional and an interprofessional practitioner. Proponents of prelicensure IPE argue that it is better to start developing an interprofessional identity before professional socialisation has fully taken hold [14]. Proponents of post licensure IPE, on the other hand, claim that having a firmly established professional identity prior to an interprofessional one gives learners greater clinical experience, confidence, and agency to advocate for the roles and responsibilities of their own profession, while also learning about other professions.

One final consideration is that wholly online learning, with its additional demands of greater self-regulated, independent learning and 'psychological distance' can be more suitable for postgraduate learners [15], who may have greater maturity and life experience to draw upon. Case studies below outline both pre and post licensure IPE considerations.

6.2.2 Teachers

Teaching OIPE is a complex, challenging, and rewarding undertaking, requiring an array of knowledge, skills and attitudes that include but go beyond those of unidisciplinary online HPE teaching, covered in Chap. 2. The heterogeneity of the OIPE cohort adds further complexity and another skillset requirement.

To begin, let's focus on what is required of an IPE teacher or educator more generally, then we'll bring in the online element. An IPE educator must be qualified and experienced in at least one health care profession but also have knowledge of a range of other professions, and experience in, and a positive attitude towards leading and facilitating interprofessional collaborative care teams and learners. Facilitation is a key skill in teaching IPE and one of the three types of teaching presence described in the Community of Inquiry Framework [2], along with direct instruction and design. Facilitation is especially important because, at its core, IPE is about enabling learners from different professions to learn with, from and about each other in order to work better together.

The list of knowledge, skills and attributes expected of an IPE facilitator is extensive. These include the following nine competencies:

- credibility in and commitment to IP education and practice,
- best practice role modelling,
- understanding of and confidence in delivering interactive learning,
- knowledge of group dynamics and use of interprofessional (and other) diversity,
- calibrating individual versus group needs and,
- conviction and good humour [16].

To this list, others add:

- knowledge of adult and experiential learning theories [17],
- conflict resolution, and,
- the ability to foster professional learners' identities [18].

OIPE teaching requires the ability to establish a learning environment in which all learners are encouraged and feel comfortable and confident to fully contribute. Essentially, an IPE teacher is not only teaching but modelling person-centred care, not merely instructing on necessary knowledge and skills but helping to transform learners into interprofessional practitioners. At the same time, they must be open to continuous learning themselves, to be both co-learners and co-teachers with their students, to model the curiosity and humility essential for effective interprofessional collaborative practice.

Finally, a 'therapeutic presence' [4] has been proposed that expands the COI model in recognition of an additional level of care and presence that may more fully support online IPE learners. Therapeutic presence is evidenced in thoughtful student-centred design, an encouraging, knowledgeable and warm 'voice' and 'tone' in written materials, assessment feedback and other general communication; regular, relevant and compassionate moderation of asynchronous discussions. It also requires skilful, inclusive facilitation of synchronous engagements such as webinars, including teamwork and enabling learners to contribute from their professional perspectives [15] and to be reflexive in their practices.

Then there are the specific capabilities required of *online* IPE teaching/facilitation, which, depending upon the level of involvement, may include:

- knowledge of online learning design principles,
- discussion moderation and synchronous webinar facilitation skills (technological and pedagogical),
- use of online tools such as breakout rooms, collaborative whiteboards, interactive polls and quizzes, videos, etc., and,
- various associated administrative responsibilities.

Issues such as lack of eye/camera alignment and audio time lag, background noise (requiring microphone muting) and varying levels of learner proficiency with online learning (both in accessing and using technology, but also 'netiquette' rules and expectations such as whether or not to have cameras on) should not be underestimated.

Co-teaching
Co-teaching or co-facilitation is a way to share workload and skillsets, and to model interprofessional collaborative practice if, as is desirable, the teachers are from different professions. There are other potential advantages associated with co-teaching, generally depending on the combination teachers, such as diversity of representation, e.g., gender, culture, seniority, profession, perspectives, etc. This allows for a dialogic facilitation approach (learning through dialogue) in webinars and skill-sharing, for example, one teacher can take a more 'technical role'.

Disadvantages of co-teaching, such as additional cost, need for alignment, reduced autonomy and risk of tension and conflict [19], are generally outweighed by the advantages, and if possible, a co-teaching, co-facilitation approach is highly recommended.

Even with co-teaching, the range of necessary knowledge, skills and attributes is considerable, and careful thought must be given to who teaches (with whom) and the training and support needed. It is recommended, therefore, that OIPE facilitators are provided with the following:

- Training in online facilitation practices and the use of online learning tools such as breakout rooms and collaborative software
- Training with a co-facilitator to establish rapport, complementary skills, division of responsibilities and a cohesive teaching approach
- Adequate time allocations to allow for considered discussion thread moderation, communication with learners and considered (co) marking and feedback of assessment tasks
- Generous time allocations to provide learners with therapeutic and social presence in addition to cognitive and teaching presence, including online office and drop in cafes.

6.3 OIPE Curriculum

What should be taught in IPE is an ongoing point of discussion, with often differing requirements and expectations between professional bodies, hospitals, and teaching institutions (including teachers and learners). **General principles of online curriculum design, outlined in Chap. 2**, apply to OPIE. However, IPE-specific curriculum considerations are detailed below.

6.3.1 IPE Frameworks

There are at least four key international IPE frameworks [20] that generally align and overlap, with minor variations in curriculum, capabilities or competencies [21–24].

We draw here upon the Interprofessional Education Collaborative's [21] four core competencies for interprofessional collaborative practice, as they encapsulate the necessary knowledge, skills and respectful, patient and relationship-centred orientation needed for effective IPCP. Paraphrased here the four core competencies of IPEC (2016) are:

- working respectfully with other professions,
- understanding one's own and other's professional roles and responsibilities to advance patient care,
- communication with patients and colleagues to support team-based patient care and,
- relationship building and team dynamics for effective patient-centred care.

Helpfully, these have been synthesised into six assessment domains by a core writing group through invitations to IPE scholars from Europe, North America, Asia, and Australia charged by the Program Committee for the 17th International Ottawa Conference on the Assessment of Competence in Medicine and the Healthcare Professions in 2016 [25], that can be further used to develop specific intended learning outcomes, targeted to the aims of a particular learning context, as discussed further below. These domains are paraphrased here as role understanding, interprofessional communication, coordination, collaborative decision-making, reflexivity, and, finally, teamwork.

6.3.2 Beyond Skills and Knowledge

IPE must go beyond the curriculum, so learners are not just acquiring skills and knowledge, i.e., "knowing that" and "knowing how" [26], but also developing capabilities, including dispositions, values, attitudes, and identities that are about ways of acting (not just knowing) in a practical context [27]. In other words, helping them *become* interprofessional practitioners.

Learning Design
As outlined earlier, there are three aspects of online teaching: design, direct instruction, and facilitation, as well as the fourth, therapeutic presence [3, 4]. We focus now on learning design as it is the foundation for the subsequent teaching and learning experience. Teaching is an art and design science, and teachers must harness and drive the use of technology for education purposes [27]. As covered in earlier chapters, we recommend a constructive alignment approach where intended learning outcomes (ILO) are carefully developed, focusing on what must be learnt rather

Fig. 6.4 Constructive alignment

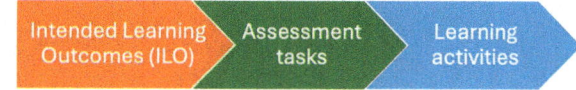

than what the topic is [28]. This informs assessments and, in turn, learning activities. Because everything derives from and is targeted toward designing learning for attaining the ILOs, it is critical that time is spent on getting them right (See Fig. 6.4).

An IPE program needs to ensure that IP specific knowledge, skills, and capabilities, such as understanding the roles and priorities of other professions in a particular clinical context such as ICU, are balanced with more generic skills like communication. Similarly, the right calibration of higher-order skills, such as *leading* an interprofessional team activity, with lower-order knowledge and skills, such as *knowing* what the advantages and disadvantages of interprofessional collaborative practice in a particular context might be. For IPE in a particular context, such as pharmacists and physicians learning to work together to dispense medication for better patient outcomes and experiences, will also likely have discipline/profession specific learning outcomes as well as those pertaining just to IPC. In the previous example, this might relate to pharmacological knowledge about the dosage of a particular medication, or synergistic effects of cytotoxic drugs, etc.

Regarding targeting the right level of learning, 'getting the verb right', is important when designing ILOs so that the appropriate level of thinking or doing to be demonstrated by the learner is clearly defined [29]. Consider, for example, whether the learner needs to explain, produce, or analyse [27]. Do they need lower-order, *recall*, or higher-order, *application, critical thinking, decision-making,* and *design*? Usually, it will be a combination of these.

There are various models to assist the ILO process:

- A revision of Bloom's taxonomy model (2001) [29]
- SOLO (Structure of the Observed Learning Outcome) taxonomy [30]
- Kirkpatrick's Typology of Educational Outcomes (1967) [31]
- Miller's Amended Pyramid (1990) [32]

Bloom's Taxonomy of Learning identifies six levels of cognitive behaviour in learning, from basic recall, through increasingly more complex and abstract thinking such as analysing, to the highest order, evaluating, and creating [30]. When developing ILOs, it is important to consider which cognitive levels are being assessed [29]. The SOLO taxonomy by Bigg and Collis [30], describe five stages of complexity of understanding, from 'pre-structural', 'uni-structural', and 'multi-structural' acquisition and reporting of information, through to 'relational' understanding of a body of knowledge, and finally to 'extended abstract' making connections and generating new knowledge. At least one ILO should aim at the highest 'extend abstract' level.

Kirkpatrick's typology [31] is a commonly used framework for designing and evaluating educational impact in IPE (See Fig. 6.5). It proposes four levels of outcome, from lower level, change in learner' reactions (1), to changes in attitudes in perceptions and attitudes and acquisition of knowledge and skills (2), to changes in

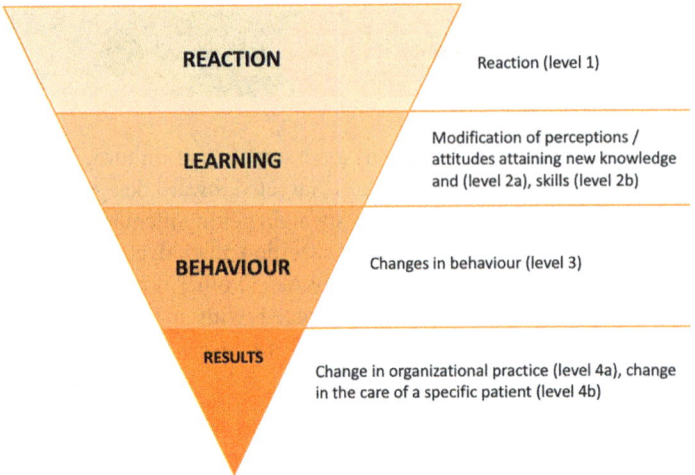

Fig. 6.5 Kirkpatrick's typology of educational outcomes

behaviour (3) and changes in organisation practice and patient care (4). The research literature consistently reports IPE participants attaining levels 1–3, but level 4 changes in practice and patient care because of IPE, although obviously desirable, are generally harder to establish.

Miller's amended pyramid [32] which aligns with and complements Kirkpatrick's typology [31], was designed specifically for assessing clinical competency in medical training but can be applied more widely to HPE and, indeed, any professional education context. The original pyramid had four levels of learning or knowledge that could be assessed, which can be summarised as knowing, knowing how (applied knowledge), showing how (demonstrated knowledge in standard context) and doing (performance in clinical practice) [33]. Miller's original pyramid has been amended to include another higher level, 'Is' (identity), as indicated in Fig. 6.6 [32].

In essence, both typologies highlight that health profession education such as IPE, requires far more than knowledge acquisition i.e. 'knowing that' and 'knowing how' [26], but also being able to apply this in a clinical context. Importantly IPE allows for development of an (inter) professional identity, demonstrating the requisite values, attitudes, beliefs, thoughts and emotions, of a practicing health (inter) professional. In other words, it can be a transformative process, not just filling a learner with knowledge and skills but changing how they think about themselves and others. This has a significant impact on what and how IPE is taught.

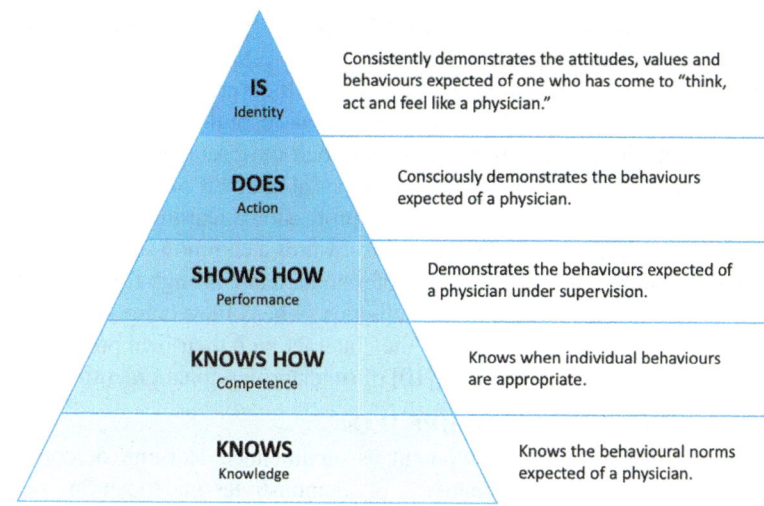

Fig. 6.6 Amended Miller's pyramid

6.3.3 Intended Learning Outcomes (ILO)

For example, using the IPEC four core competencies [21] and focusing on 'communication' in the context of palliative care, intended learning outcomes could be that learners will be able to:

- begin engaging in conversations around death with patient and their families, or,
- discuss a patient's end-of-life preferences with colleagues.

Alternatively, focusing on 'relationship building and team dynamics' could result in intended learning outcomes such as learners will be able to:

- initiate an interprofessional team conversation about a patient's discharge, or,
- design and implement a strategy to resolve conflict in an interprofessional team conflict scenario.

Identities

> "Learning transforms who we are and what we can do, it is an experience of identity. It is not just an accumulation of skills and information, but a process of becoming…" [34].

Identities are complex, multiple, relational, and dynamic. OIPE learners come with multiple identities, such as professionals, (co) learners and interprofessional collaborators. These multiple identities are developed, shaped, affirmed or reflected in relationship to synchronous and asynchronous interactions with others. Our stories of self-identity echo, reverberate, distort, or dissipate in response to feedback from others, including peers and teachers. This, in turn, affects confidence, agency and practice. In post-licensure IPE, learners with pre-established professional identities may more readily represent and advocate for their profession's roles, responsibilities, and priorities, providing potentially more authentic interprofessional learning interactions for all learners. However, their uni-professional education and experience may also have entrenched stereotypes about their own and other professions that are difficult to undo and limit interprofessional learning. Allowing learners to engage in non-hierarchical interactions towards a common superordinate goal [1], such as learning to work in an interprofessional team through formal and informal, synchronous, and asynchronous activities, where they come to understand more about other professions, and how they interact with their own profession, can help them develop the 'dual identity' [10] of (inter)professional practitioner.

Recommendations for Creating OIPE ILOs
- Consider including IPE development as an intended learning outcome, e.g. 'reflects upon professional identity… or 'demonstrates understanding of other professions roles, responsibilities and priorities…
- Create opportunities for informal social interactions through dedicated online cafés and asynchronous discussions
- Interprofessional group activities and assessment
- Provide feedback on IP specifically
- Reflection through journaling on the process of interprofessional interaction, not just the product
- Reflection on professional and interprofessional identity (metacognition)
- Consider use of IP metrics for learner self-assessment, pre and post education to measure learning

6.4 OIPE Pedagogy

How IPE is taught and learnt is as important as *what* is taught and learnt, because much of the IPE learning occurs through peer learning with, from and about each other, facilitated by teachers, rather than through direct instruction. Maintaining focus on the learner, there are multiple pedagogical elements to consider when designing an OIPE program, including:

- duration,
- sequencing and pacing,
- synchronous and asynchronous engagement,
- individual and group activities (including assessment),
- didactic versus experiential, activity and/or case-based learning, and,
- clinical/work-integrated learning.

Which of these elements is used and how are likewise dependent on various factors such as existing logistical constraints, e.g., time, learner cohort, level of technical and design support, intended learning outcomes, teacher knowledge, skills, availability, and support, etc.

Pedagogical Theories

Key theories which underpin online education were previously summarised in Chap. 1. Four of these that are particularly relevant to OIPE are:

- Knowles four principles of adult learning (andragogy) highlight the importance of including self-planned, relevant, experiential, and problem-centred learning [35].
- Laurillard outlines six types of learning that can occur via digital technology: acquisition, inquiry, practice, production and discussion, and collaboration [27].
- Schön posits not just problem *solving* but problem *setting*. Reflective practice includes both reflection *in* action and reflection *on* action, leading to insight into one's implicit knowledge and learning from experience [36].
- Finally, the Community of Inquiry model provides a conceptual framework that identifies the three types of presence, cognitive, social and teaching, for a successful educational experience [2].

In combination, elements of these theories can be used to help design and deliver successful OIPE, which:

- allow learners to bring problems (clinical cases) from their own work practices to use as class case discussions,
- use experiential and problem-based activities and assessments, with sufficient didactic learning to contextualise the learning,
- ensure activities, including assessments are interprofessional collaboration-based, i.e., group assessments, whenever possible and appropriate (including peer feedback on process),
- embed reflectivity and reflexivity into learning through journaling, discussions, and assessments,
- build in opportunities for interprofessional social interactions (for informal conversations not necessarily program-related) in both synchronous and asynchronous engagement, and
- ensure consistent teaching presence in both asynchronous (discussions, assessment feedback, self-recorded videos, emails and announcements, etc) and synchronous through webinars, online 'open-office' hours, etc.

6.4.1 How Long Does an OIPE Program Need to Be?

The duration of formal OIPE can be anything from a focused 2-hr online module to a 2-year master's degree course. There is little evidence on the ideal duration to achieve learning across the six assessment domains [25], let alone to fully develop the necessary 'dual identity' [10]. The Contact hypothesis [1] would suggest that the longer the duration of contact, up to a certain point, the greater the opportunity to gain an understanding of and break down stereotypes about an outgroup, i.e., other professions. Where that 'certain point' is, however, has yet to be established. IPE is not an exact science and should be ongoing, with practitioners continually open to new learning.

When considering duration, it is not just a question of how much time is spent over what period, but how that time is spent, synchronous or asynchronous, pacing, sequencing, intensity, and volume of learning activities, etc. Somewhat unhelpfully, we can only recommend that OIPE be as long as necessary to achieve the intended learning outcomes within any existing constraints, such as resource allocation, teacher and learner availability, existing course structure, timetabling, and term/semester length, etc. Pacing and sequencing and balance of synchronous and asynchronous delivery should also be considered as discussed in earlier chapters.

6.4.2 OIPE Discussion Threads

Discussion threads may seem like an obvious, unexciting, and 'lo-fi' learning activity (low fidelity, simplified, or minimalistic learning activity), but this is to underestimate their pedagogical power. If designed well with timely and thoughtful teaching presence through regular and meaningful moderation, they are a highly effective mode of interprofessional learning. Case study 1 below, shows that Discussions provided the structural spine that integrated most of the pedagogical design elements from the learning theories above. This included real-life case scenarios that learners could reflect upon, consider, and discuss from their own professional perspectives without the pressure of having to think on their feet, negotiate professional status hierarchies, or other pressures of in-person or synchronous online environments.

If designed with appropriate rules of engagement and prompts, Discussions also create a safe space for learners to practice proffering professional opinions, explain clinical reasoning and decision making, respectfully disagree, and negotiate points of tension in their own time. These written contributions can be more well thought out and articulated than off-the-cuff verbal comments made in real-time. Furthermore, as this is 'captured' in text, as well as constraining the extent of any tension and conflict, it allows for later review and reflection.

When setting up discussion threads, consider the following:

- Go for quality over quantity, e.g., one or two weekly prompts (see below) that facilitate authentic participation. Dividing larger classes into smaller discussion groups can mitigate against unwieldy discussions and engineer specific interprofessional groupings.
- Establish clear parameters so that learners are not compelled to respond just for the sake of it and are clear about what, how (much) and when they are expected to contribute.

- Require a professional tone (but not necessarily an academic one). Frame it more as a clinical simulation or virtual MDTM than an academic exercise.
- Consider assigning a small mark/grade weighting to signal the learning importance of discussions.
- Discussions may be assessed for consistent and relevant contributions but also a reflection on a salient example and/or a summary of 'best contributions'.
- Establish teaching presence (but do not over-impose) through consistent and constructive moderation [27]. Correct, probe, prompt, and challenge but model positivity towards inclusive interprofessional interactions [37].
- Vary the types of discussions, such as case studies, that allow learners to contribute their professional knowledge and perspectives, prompt questions that elicit clinical reasoning, problem-solving (and setting) and decision-making, and/or raise moral and ethical dilemmas. These generate opportunities to exercise higher-order skills such as critiquing and negotiating, rather than simple fact-type questions which require a specific answer (which can be done through quizzes if necessary), leaving no room for further discussion.
- Invite learners to contribute cases from their own clinical practices for discussion in simulated MDTMs (with appropriate privacy considerations).
- More creative use of discussions might include asynchronous role plays, where learners may take the part of another profession in a given scenario, and collaborative narrative-based activities, such as collectively writing a story of a patient's perceptions and experiences of interprofessional care. These types of activities can elicit important IPCP skills such as perspective-taking and empathy.

6.4.3 Synchronous Web-Based Video in OIPE

Using web-based video platforms such as Teams and Zoom is now commonplace in online and blended learning, even more so since COVID-19 and the rapid transition to online learning. There are opportunities to innovate and avoid the outdated 60–90 min 'stand and deliver' lectures online.

When designing OIPE, an important early consideration is to decide whether there will be any webinars and, if so, how many, when and of what sort. This will depend on various factors, including teacher availability and resourcing, but most importantly, the duration of the program. Although some type of synchronous engagement is recommended in any form of OIPE, it is of particular importance in longer-duration OIPE programs, such as those within the traditional academic term or semester-long programs that run over several months.

Webinars are beneficial in OIPE for several reasons, including:

- enabling real-time interactions that are closer to 'real life' with some of its visual and paralinguistic cues,
- simulating clinical practices such as telehealth and virtual MDTMS,
- helping pace learning as a synchronous touchpoint,

- enhancing collective cohort experience and,
- enabling a greater teaching presence and allowing for immediate sense checking and Q&A on things such as assessment.

There are also some drawbacks to webinars, namely that depending upon learners' locations, time zones and work commitments, scheduling can be difficult. To get around this, webinars can be made non-compulsory and recorded for those who cannot attend live. However, this can further reduce live attendance, just as lecture recordings do for in-person learning. A key benefit of synchronous engagement is the immediacy of communication, greater verisimilitude, i.e., giving the appearance of being true or real, and live presence with teachers and peers that allows not only for cognitive engagement but informal and ad-hoc social interactions, which, while not the same, come close to approximating real-life interactions. Ideally, depending on duration and teacher availability, a regular weekly or fortnightly webinar to maintain pacing and presence is recommended.

6.4.4 Types of Webinars

Given the wide range of possible formats and pedagogical and curricular options, the next consideration is what types of webinars to use. Options include:

- online lecture, which (in abridged format) can allow learners to access experts and clinical contexts not otherwise possible,
- web tutorials, e.g. tutor led oral discussions, Q & As on learning topics and assessment tasks,
- student presentations, critical debates, role plays, and clinical simulations such as multidisciplinary team meetings.
- learner assessment, summative as well as formative, through observation of tasks, such as presentation or clinical scenarios, or viva questioning formats.
- 'open-office' webinars, providing one-on-one access to teaching staff to discuss learning and progress and,
- informal online cafés, e.g., dedicated student-only Zoom or Teams link, allowing learners to drop in for informal social interactions with peers.

While the above options apply to online learning generally, some can be adapted to particular advantage for OIPE. The many possible variations of the web-tutorial provide increased opportunities for learners to engage with other professions and to learn with, from and about them. Learning can be 'scaffolded' through lead up activities, such as asynchronous discussions on a particular scenario, that can help prepare learners for the pressure of real-time interactions. This is where the teacher as facilitator comes to the fore, setting the scene and rules of engagement, and ensuring a psychologically safe space for all learners, while not imposing themselves too much, letting learners interact and resolve tensions, disagreements, and conflicts by themselves as much as possible. Outright conflict is rare, particularly with marks/grades at stake and a teacher present, but subtle power dynamics and micro-aggressions are more common and must be dealt with promptly but sensitively to avoid escalation and emotional harm. As these will generally replicate and reinforce the types of status issues and dynamics that arise in IPCP, they present teachable moments and with appropriate handling, including debriefing, can provide excellent real world interprofessional learning opportunities.

6.4.5 Webinar Rules of Engagement

Key to effective webinars is establishing clear ground rules. Some of these are standard and the consequences of serious infringements in respect of privacy, or inappropriate behaviour will be stated in enrolment. To create a trusted environment that encourages learners to openly share their professional experiences and perspectives, for the benefit of all, a clear policy of anonymisation of any patient details, is essential. It is also highly recommended that The Chatham House Rule[1] is enforced, which states "When a meeting, or part thereof, is held under the Chatham House Rule, participants are free to use the information received, but neither the identity nor the affiliation of the speaker(s), nor that of any other participant, may be revealed".

Although it should go without saying, the need for courteous and respectful interactions is particularly important in IPE and should always be reinforced by teachers. Some rules fall into the category of 'netiquette', i.e., they suggest attitudes and behaviours that improve the experience of all learners. Be clear about simple things like muting when not speaking, raising the hand icon to indicate a desire to speak, and having your camera on where possible, as this can facilitate greater engagement and enhance the teaching and learning experience (this should not be mandated as there are valid reasons for not doing so, e.g., concerns about privacy and not wanting to reveal location, poor internet connection that prevents stable video, self-consciousness, etc). All participants should be encouraged to contribute, but not coerced, as the aim is to create an environment where everyone feels that they can speak up when they have something to say. Conversely, frequent contributors must learn not to dominate to make space for others. (Listening is a highly undervalued clinical communication skill.) These can take some time and one of the benefits of having regular webinars with the same participants is that they develop familiarity and confidence, and rhythms of interaction are established, just as with IPCP teams.

Further suggestions for webinars include:

- Provide prior activities that prepare learners to get the most from the webinar such as reading patient cases to be discussed, e.g., Flipped classroom approach
- Use breakout rooms to create opportunities for smaller group interactions

---

[1] https://www.chathamhouse.org/about-us/chatham-house-rule

- Co-facilitation of webinars is highly recommended
- Try Gamification-Team-building skills (e.g. escape rooms)
- Make use of tools such as collaborative whiteboards, bulletin boards as well as quizzes and polls, etc., to enliven learning
- Give opportunities for learners to co-facilitate sessions

6.4.6 Virtual MDTMs

A common site of interprofessional collaborative practice is the multidisciplinary team meeting (MDTM). Although described as multidisciplinary, if done well, they are interprofessional, as different professions (and disciplines) collaborate for the common goal of better patient outcomes. Unfortunately, given the time pressure, professional status and hierarchies of MDTMs, typically led by a senior physician or surgeon, can also be sites of tension and displays of power and even conflict.

There is an opportunity in OIPE to create synchronous learning experiences that accurately simulate virtual multidisciplinary team meetings and help to develop best practices. For example, a webinar with a case-based focus, facilitated by the teacher who acts as the meeting chair and invites respectful, non-hierarchical contributions from all professional perspectives and within a reasonable timeframe, could model an ideal MDTM scenario. Alternatively, the teacher could create more 'realistic' MDTMs by introducing time pressures and 'turning up the heat' to simulate a more stressful situation. Conflict resolution techniques could then be modelled, and a full debrief could allow learners to reflect on how they reacted, how others reacted and what they think might have done differently.

6.5 Assessment

OIPE presents an opportunity to do assessments differently and to move beyond the traditional essay, exam and MCQ approach, although acknowledging concerns of resourcing, standardisation, and scale. Indeed, in some respects, OIPE necessitates a more innovative and creative approach. The types, amount, and weighting of assessment in an OIPE are contingent on the nature of the program and, specifically, the intended learning outcomes. As described above, these may be solely and primarily interprofessional focused, or they may be integrated with another substantive topic within which the interprofessional education takes place, for example, cancer care. Either way, the assessments must enable learners to receive regular, timely and constructive feedback that benchmarks and guides their ongoing interprofessional development.

6.5.1 Assessing What?

The first consideration should, therefore, be, what is being assessed? In straightforward terms, what is it that we want the learner to demonstrate they can know, do or be? This should be decided from the outset in the careful design of the intended learning outcomes, detailing the type and level of thinking, doing and being that is expected. Each assessment task requires demonstration of one or more of the learning outcomes, i.e., an individual task does not need to cover all ILOs, but the overall suite of assessment will need to do so, and some ILOs may be covered in more than one task.

6.5.2 Pacing, Sequencing and Weighting

Next, consider the number of assessment tasks, pacing and sequencing, i.e., when they occur in the program, in what order, and their respective weightings. Programs within existing academic courses should have clear guidelines about assessment, including word equivalence or time-based parameters for weighting and when they should occur, but this is not an exact science.

The general principles of formative and summative assessments and the need to provide learners with regular, timely and meaningful feedback, *of*, *for*, and *about* learning is of particular importance in OIPE. It is good practice to provide feedback early on in a program with a relatively lower-weighted task to establish confidence and a baseline, assess again around the middle of the program and finish with a higher-weighted task at the end of the teaching period. These should also be structured so that each task builds upon the learning and feedback of the previous task, and for learning purposes (although this is not a popular sentiment), the feedback is generally more important than the mark given.

6.5.3 Peer Feedback and Group Assessment

In OIPE, where learning is as much about the *process* of working together interprofessionally as it is about an end *product*, this should be reflected in how the learners are assessed.

To this end, group assessments and peer-reviewed assessments play a vital role in OIPE, not the least because they signal that the process of learning and working together is key. At least one assessment task in an OIPE program should, therefore, be a group assessment task that requires the application of aspects of authentic interprofessional collaborative practice. Ideally, these will require learners to *do*, i.e., role play their own (or another) profession in a realistic scenario, such as contributing to a particular case in an online MDTM and then reflecting upon the process and the nature of the interactions, what they learnt and recommendations for improvement. This reflective component could be an individual or group written piece or presentation.

The second aspect of this is peer-review/feedback and/ or marking (grading), which can be done with individual as well as group assessment. Peer feedback, rather than peer marking, is of greater benefit in OIPE and learning to critique and *give* constructive feedback should be part of an assessment (rather than peer feedback being factored into the recipient's mark/feedback). In a group task, peer feedback should reflect upon and analyse the IP process and be assessed on the quality of the insights, degree of learning shown, and constructive suggestions provided by the learner.

6.5.4 Reflection

Given the aim of OIPE, to help learners develop their professional and interprofessional (dual) identities, a reflective component to the assessment is essential. This reinforces the importance of ongoing reflective interprofessional practice and how learning may alter or affirm their professional and interprofessional identities and their confidence and sense of agency. Another opportunity in OIPE is to create authentic, work-integrated assessment tasks informed by, and in turn, informing the learner's own clinical practices. This may involve learner-initiated assessment tasks or projects that allow them to target their learning to be specifically relevant and applicable for their own clinical context.

6.5.5 Rubrics

While not a silver bullet, a well-constructed rubric (assessment matrix or grading scheme), that clearly outlines expectations, and the specific criteria that are being assessed, the weighting (percentage values of marks for each criterion) and the evaluative ranges e.g. unsatisfactory, satisfactory, good, very good, excellent etc., of each, can help teachers and learners be clear about what the explicit aims of the assessment are. Although rubrics take time to set up initially, they can help the learner achieve the intended learning outcomes more fairly and help teachers mark more efficiently and consistently.

A good rubric design for online HPE, includes assessment criteria and indicators that are accurately defined and described, meeting the ILOs and with an assessment scale that is logical, reasonable and allows for nuanced mark allocation and feedback. There are many open-source rubric guides and templates available online, including the Interprofessional Collaborator Assessment Rubric (ICAR), by the National Center for Interprofessional Practice and Education [38].

Important considerations for rubrics in OIPE include:

- Process outcome criteria about not just what was achieved but how
- Criteria that relate to the four core competencies and six domains of IPCP outlined in 6.3.1 IPE Frameworks
- Criteria on reflection including on own and other professions
- Balancing 'higher and lower order' knowledge and skills, outlined in 6.3.2 Beyond skills and knowledge
- Fully differentiated criteria and value descriptors

> **Case Study 1: A Wholly Online Postgraduate master's Course**
> Why: To improve the oncology-specific knowledge and skills of healthcare professionals to meet an increasing workforce demand and ultimately to improve the outcomes of people with cancer. To fill the gap in online, multidisciplinary cancer-care focused postgraduate education [39].
>
> How: A wholly online Master of Cancer Sciences (MCS) program with an industry-led curriculum and using asynchronous and synchronous engagement with strong teaching presence in both discussions and webinars. Students complete eight subjects, four core and four electives. This includes a research project (See Fig. 6.7).
>
> The Course purports to be multidisciplinary rather than interprofessional, but student feedback and research suggest that they perceived and experienced extensive interprofessional learning with, from and about each other [40].

> **Case Study 2: A Short Course in Interprofessional Digital Health**
> Why: To foster skilled interdisciplinary learning communities and digital health champions who can work collaboratively to solve complex problems using Learning Health Systems (LHS).
>
> How: A 13-week wholly online short course in interprofessional working groups of five members who learned together, sharing experiences and perspectives. A flipped classroom approach used various collaborative eLearning tools for mind mapping, data interrogation, visualisation, and interpretation, clinical process modelling software, and a virtual digital care platform for prototyping digital health solutions (See Fig. 6.8).
>
> Learners found the course engaging and useful, increasing perceived confidence and creating common understanding and language for interprofessional interactions and use of digital health technologies. Some identified as leaders in the area, post-course. [41].

What's Next?

There is still a long way we can take OIPE with existing technology through improvements in pedagogy. However, the future is already here, and technological

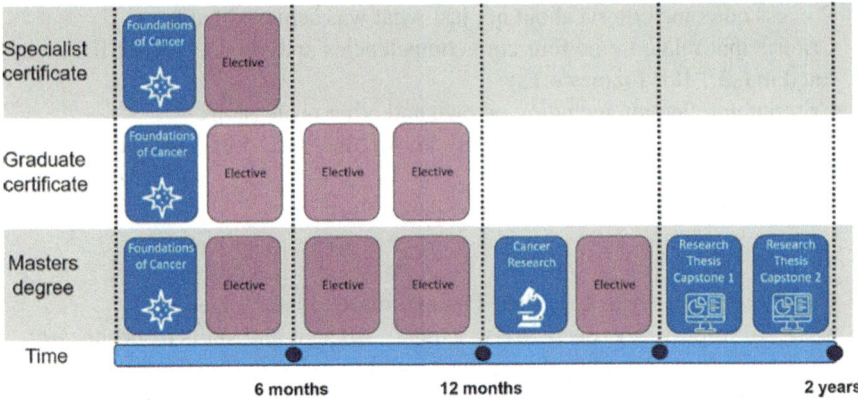

Fig. 6.7 Nested structure of the Master of Cancer Sciences (Case study 1). Source [39]

advancements in the areas of AI, AR, and VR are creating new challenges and opportunities, as discussed in Chaps. 4 and 7 of this manual. In these chapters, we briefly explore the vast potential of technological and pedagogical advancements to enhance OIPE, along with some of the red flags and risks.

- AI-generated OSCE patients
- VR simulations of IP interactions with colleagues and patients
- Use of data from learner analytics to map IPE interactions
- Use of AI for teacher/student assessment interactions

6.6 Tips and Tricks

- When planning and designing OIPE think specifically about why you are doing it, who it is for (which specific professions and levels) and where the learning will happen e.g., classroom, clinic, computer?
- Intentionally design for specific interprofessional learning outcomes, i.e., don't just assume they will happen. Include not just IP skills and knowledge but identity formation.
- Include activities that require interprofessional collaboration through both synchronous and asynchronous engagements, including assessments e.g., case discussions in MDTs.
- Design 'two-way' work integrated activities that encourage learners to apply IPE learning in clinical contexts and bring their experiences back into shared learning.
- Prioritise teaching presence and include therapeutic presence (as well as design, direct instruction and facilitation) to model learner/patient-centred practice
- Use interprofessional team teaching whenever possible to model IP practice and enhance the learning and teaching experience.

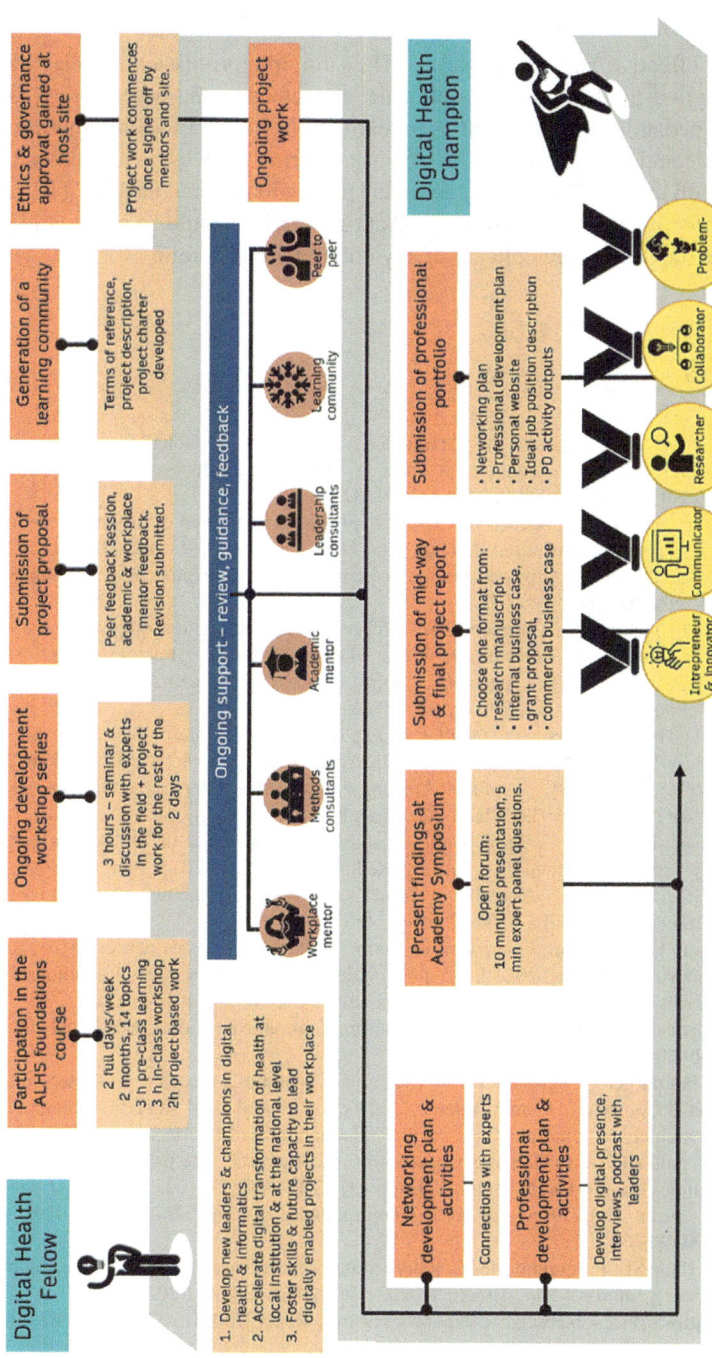

Fig. 6.8 Learning Health Systems (Case study 2). Source [41]

6.7 Conclusion

OIPE is an effective way of preparing HPEs for interprofessional collaborative practice. Beyond the basic benefits of scale, convenience and accessibility, OIPE offers other pedagogical opportunities to learn, with, from and about other professions in a safe and supported way. As well as acquiring knowledge and skills it can also assist with the development of the (inter) professional 'dual identity' [10], necessary for effective IPCP. Therefore, integration of OIPE should be an integral consideration in the design and delivery of any online HPE program.

References

1. Allport GW. The nature of prejudice [internet]. Doubleday; 1958. [cited 2024 Jun 27]. Available from: https://research.ebsco.com/linkprocessor/plink?id=7ee06695-b237-399b-9a1d-eb811981e37d
2. Garrison DR, Anderson T, Archer W. Critical inquiry in a text-based environment: computer conferencing in higher education. Int High Educ [Internet]. 1999;2(2–3):87–105. [cited 2024 Jun 27]. Available from: https://research.ebsco.com/linkprocessor/plink?id=29f0299b-37b8-3e7f-8059-2c9c00afb06e
3. Anderson T, Rourke L, Garrison DR, Archer W. Assessing teaching presence in a computer conferencing context. J Async Learn Network [Internet]. 2001;5(2):1. [cited 2024 Jun 28]. Available from: https://research.ebsco.com/linkprocessor/plink?id=cc50d82f-8ef6-3d37-9ccb-eb673a2d1e45
4. Bluteau P. The good enough facilitator: exploring online interprofessional therapeutic facilitation in times of COVID-19. J Interprof Care [Internet]. 2020;34(5):647–54. [cited 2024 Jun 28]. Available from: https://research.ebsco.com/linkprocessor/plink?id=776f21a6-2133-3933-af7c-0dd0eda5c9a1
5. Bodenheimer T, Sinsky C. From triple to quadruple aim: care of the patient requires care of the provider. Annals of Family Medicine [Internet] 2014 Nov 1 [cited 2024 Jun 27];12(6):573–6. Available from: https://research.ebsco.com/linkprocessor/plink?id=2f8e8c6f-a9cb-32ba-9263-e26a5aac14a6
6. World Health Organization. Framework for action on interprofessional education and collaborative practice 2010; [cited 2024 Jun 27] Available from: https://www.who.int/publications/i/item/framework-for-action-on-interprofessional-education-collaborative-practice
7. CAIPE. The centre for the advancement of interprofessional education. 2017; [cited 2024 Jun 27] Available from: https://www.caipe.org/
8. Amichai-Hamburger Y, McKenna KYA. The contact hypothesis reconsidered: interacting via the Internet. J Comp-Med Comm [Internet]. 2006;11(3) [cited 2024 Jun 27]. Available from: https://research.ebsco.com/linkprocessor/plink?id=aad6b659-db18-31b5-8b75-a387892ae88a
9. Hean S, Craddock D, O'Halloran C. Learning theories and interprofessional education: a user's guide. Learn Health Soc Care [Internet]. 2009;8(4):250–62. [cited 2024 Jun 27]. Available from: https://research.ebsco.com/linkprocessor/plink?id=4879b910-0103-3b96-9823-10c0f908b172
10. Khalili H, Price SL. From uniprofessionality to interprofessionality: dual vs dueling identities in healthcare. J Interprof Care [Internet]. 2022;36(3):473–8. [cited 2024 Jun 27]. Available from: https://research.ebsco.com/linkprocessor/plink?id=223de1f3-f34e-320a-8894-1d2c712c02ee

11. Latour B. Reassembling the social: an introduction to actor-network-theory [internet]. Oxford University Press; 2005. [cited 2024 Jun 28]. Available from: https://research.ebsco.com/linkprocessor/plink?id=c17832a5-857e-3461-a094-7aa3c017ac3f
12. Hammick M, Freeth D, Koppel I, Reeves S, Barr H. A best evidence systematic review of interprofessional education: BEME Guide no. 9. Med Teacher [Internet]. 2007;29(8):735–51. [cited 2024 Jun 28]. Available from: https://research.ebsco.com/linkprocessor/plink?id=b87e3a57-0fb6-34a0-ba91-b0666a2b7ffb
13. Kok D, Dushyanthen S, Peters G, Sapkaroski D, Barrett M, Sim J, et al. Virtual reality and augmented reality in radiation oncology education–A review and expert commentary. 2022. [cited 2024 Jun 28]; Available from: https://research.ebsco.com/linkprocessor/plink?id=9b175477-a550-3c47-a47e-2ad61786b660
14. Areskog NH. The need for multiprofessional health education in undergraduate studies. Med Educ [Internet]. 1988;22(4):251–2. [cited 2024 Jun 28]. Available from: https://research.ebsco.com/linkprocessor/plink?id=aa56dff2-a8c9-3674-9f22-b5a36fda2222
15. Solomon P, King S. Online interprofessional education: perceptions of faculty facilitators. J Phys Therapy Educ (American Physical Therapy Association, Education Section) [Internet]. 2010;24(1):51–3. [cited 2024 Jun 28]. Available from: https://research.ebsco.com/linkprocessor/plink?id=347309b0-036d-3ec6-b08b-b0113c54beae
16. Freeth D, Reeves S, Koppel I, Hammick M, Barr H. Evaluating interprofessional education: a self-help guide. In: UK Higher education academy learning and teaching support network for health sciences and practice. London: Wiley; 2005. [cited 2024 Jun 28]; https://doi.org/Occasionalpaperno5.
17. Hall P, Weaver L. Interdisciplinary education and teamwork: a long and winding road. Med Educ [Internet]. 2001;35(9):867–75. [cited 2024 Jun 28]. Available from: https://research.ebsco.com/linkprocessor/plink?id=9a63b5bc-fc2a-36a3-9cab-d6849e18f5c3
18. Davoli GW, Fine L-J. Stacking the deck for success in interprofessional collaboration. Health Promo Pract [Internet]. 2004;5(3):266–70. [cited 2024 Jun 28]. Available from: https://research.ebsco.com/linkprocessor/plink?id=4ecf5a9f-f05e-386c-ac89-1ec50e5695ee
19. Crow J, Smith L. Using co-teaching as a means of facilitating interprofessional collaboration in health and social care. J Interprof Care [Internet]. 2003;17(1):45–55. [cited 2024 Jun 28]. Available from: https://research.ebsco.com/linkprocessor/plink?id=9346163f-c1a9-36cb-b9f8-e720248a829f
20. Thistlethwaite JE, Forman D, Matthews LR, Rogers GD, Steketee C, Yassine T. Competencies and frameworks in interprofessional education: a comparative analysis. Acad Med [Internet]. 2014;89(6):869–75. [cited 2024 Jun 28]. Available from: https://research.ebsco.com/linkprocessor/plink?id=19519784-87b2-3bfd-9b40-921993df3f9a
21. Interprofessional Education Collaborative Expert Panel. Core competencies for interprofessional collaborative practice: 2016 update. Washington, DC: Interprofessional Education Collaborative [Internet]; 2016. [cited 2024 Jun 28]. Available from: https://ipec.memberclicks.net/assets/2016-Update.pdf
22. Walsh CL, Gordon MF, Marshall M, Wilson F, Hunt T. Interprofessional capability: a developing framework for interprofessional education. Nurse Educ Pract [Internet]. 2005;5(4):230–7. [cited 2024 Jun 28]. Available from: https://research.ebsco.com/linkprocessor/plink?id=79a34166-3344-3f34-9688-eb6567ecc44e
23. Canadian Interprofessional Health Collaborative. A national interprofessional competency framework [Internet]. 2010; [cited 2024 Jun 28]. Available from: www.cihc.ca/files/CIHC_IPCompetencies_Feb1210.pdf
24. Gum LF, Lloyd A, Lawn S, Richards JN, Lindemann I, Sweet L, et al. Developing an interprofessional capability framework for teaching healthcare students in a primary healthcare setting. J Interprof Care [Internet]. 2013;27(6):454–60. [cited 2024 Jun 28]. Available from: https://research.ebsco.com/linkprocessor/plink?id=d5adbc30-51db-3a90-ae43-6a02ba9f0cbb
25. Rogers GD, Thistlethwaite JE, Anderson ES, Abrandt Dahlgren M, Grymonpre RE, Moran M, et al. International consensus statement on the assessment of interprofessional learning out-

comes. Med Teacher [Internet]. 2017;39(4):347–59. [cited 2024 Jun 28]. Available from: https://research.ebsco.com/linkprocessor/plink?id=01b72e9a-0576-3869-b9d3-24ba98a64772
26. Ryle G. Knowing how and knowing that: the presidential address. Proc Aristotelian Soc [Internet]. 1945;46:1–16. [cited 2024 Jun 28]. Available from: https://research.ebsco.com/linkprocessor/plink?id=964d172d-324a-37ec-b22b-e2cbca00ab52
27. Laurillard D. Teaching as a design science: building pedagogical patterns for learning and technology [Internet]. Routledge. –2012. [cited 2024 Jun 28]. Available from: https://research.ebsco.com/linkprocessor/plink?id=e16d28b6-7bdc-3def-a048-aee598128c11
28. Biggs J, Tang, C. Constructive alignment: An outcomes-based approach to teaching anatomy. In: Chan, L., Pawlina, W. (Eds.), Teaching anatomy. Springer, Cham. 2015 https://doi.org/10.1007/978-3-319-08930-0_4
29. Krathwohl DR. A revision of bloom's taxonomy: an overview. Theory Pract [Internet]. 2002;41(4):212–8. [cited 2024 Jun 28] Available from: https://research.ebsco.com/linkprocessor/plink?id=bae16f24-377c-3c29-8bce-76be771f7aa2
30. Biggs JB. Evaluating the quality of learning: the SOLO taxonomy (structure of the observed learning outcome) [Internet]. Academic; 1982. [cited 2024 Jun 28]. Available from: https://research.ebsco.com/linkprocessor/plink?id=8f2e01a0-ce1d-3fbe-a0b9-2f75579cffc2
31. Kirkpatrick D. Evaluation of training. In: Craig R, Bittel L, editors. Training and development handbook. New York: McGraw-Hill; 1967. p. 131–67. [cited 2024 Jun 28].
32. Cruess RL, Cruess SR, Steinert Y. Amending Miller's pyramid to include professional identity formation. Acad Med [Internet]. 2016;91(2):180–5. [cited 2024 Jun 28]. Available from: https://research.ebsco.com/linkprocessor/plink?id=8a548c6c-4229-317d-bdb1-3a45abc63c84
33. Witheridge A, Ferns G, Scott-Smith W. Revisiting Miller's pyramid in medical education: the gap between traditional assessment and diagnostic reasoning. Int J Med Educ [Internet]. 2019;10:191–2. [cited 2024 Jun 29]. Available from: https://research.ebsco.com/linkprocessor/plink?id=8f61ed64-60fe-323e-bb54-e4ccc1f84af2
34. Wenger E. Communities of practice: learning, meaning, and identity [internet]. Cambridge University Press; 1998. [cited 2024 Jun 29]. Available from: https://research.ebsco.com/linkprocessor/plink?id=2c19f0c2-845c-3fc9-8c39-647fd1bba714
35. Knowles MS. Andragogy in action. Applying modern principles of adult education. San Francisco, CA: Jossey Bass; 1984. [cited 2024 Jun 29]
36. Schön DA. The reflective practitioner: how professionals think in action [internet]. Routledge; 2016. [cited 2024 Jun 29]. Available from: https://research.ebsco.com/linkprocessor/plink?id=6b394b51-b46f-311c-ac0c-c8b17b0d6d0b
37. Dallimore EJ, Hertenstein JH, Platt MB. Classroom participation and discussion effectiveness: student-generated strategies. Comm Educ [Internet]. 2004;53(1):1. Available from: https://research.ebsco.com/linkprocessor/plink?id=4f877ad6-450b-3cb4-8ebf-a124a6b18875
38. Interprofessional Collaborator Assessment Rubric (ICAR) [Internet]. National center for interprofessional practice and education. 2016. Available from: https://nexusipe.org/advancing/assessment-evaluation/interprofessional-collaborator-assessment-rubric-icar
39. Lai-Kwon J, Dushyanthen S, Seignior D, Barrett M, Buisman-Pijlman F, Buntine A, et al. Designing a wholly online, multidisciplinary master of cancer sciences degree. BMC Med Educ [Internet]. 2023. Jul 31 [cited 2024 Jun 30]. Available from: https://research.ebsco.com/linkprocessor/plink?id=1e4cebda-add7-32f0-9edf-8eaa9fecd548;23:544.
40. Seignior D. The student experience of online interprofessional education in cancer sciences: a philosophical-empirical inquiry. Doctor of Education. University of Melbourne; 2024. Accessed July 1, 2024, from https://minerva-access.unimelb.edu.au/items/eed25bf0-b581-4d5b-a9cf-c02a3bcb3e0f
41. Dushyanthen S, Perrier M, Chapman W, Layton M, Lyons K. Fostering the use of learning health systems through a fellowship program for interprofessional clinicians. Learn Health Syst [Internet]. 2022;6(4) Available from: https://research.ebsco.com/linkprocessor/plink?id=1dcc7b35-78fd-3711-9bc5-1a259f4da9c4

Chapter 7
Applications of Artificial Intelligence to Health Professional Education

Thomas Cochrane, David Seignior, and David L. Kok

Abstract The utility of Artificial Intelligence (AI) in online Health Professional Education (HPE) has come to the fore with the release of publicly accessible online generative AI (GenAI) interfaces. The result has been an exponential increase in the use of these digital tools in HPE design and delivery. In this chapter, we outline current and emerging applications of AI in digital HPE contexts, divided into three major categories:

1. Opportunities for AI to aid in the design and delivery of HPE programs
2. Risks and vulnerabilities that AI poses to health professional educational methods
3. Necessity to integrate AI competencies into HPE curricula

Ethical implications of AI use in HPE are also discussed as they form a key consideration for any educator. Finally, a basic roadmap of institutional and professional responses to AI in digital health education are outlined to help educators be best positioned to effectively and constructively utilise this game-changing new technology in their own context.

Key Points
- GenAI has the capability to assist/supplement health professional educators in many aspects of educational curriculum design and delivery.
- AI has exposed a number of risks and vulnerabilities of current health professional educational methods—particularly in assessment. Hence, many assessments would benefit from being reconsidered in light of AI to mitigate against its misuse.
- Incorporation of AI competencies into HPE curricula is critical to equip graduates with the capabilities to critically use these tools in practice.

T. Cochrane · D. Seignior
University of Melbourne, Melbourne, Australia

D. L. Kok (✉)
University of Melbourne, Melbourne, Australia

Peter MacCallum Cancer Centre, Melbourne, Australia
e-mail: dkok@unimelb.edu.au

© The Author(s), under exclusive license to Springer Nature Switzerland AG 2025
D. L. Kok et al. (eds.), *Best Practices in Online Education*, IAMSE Manuals, https://doi.org/10.1007/978-3-031-90349-6_7

- AI requires professional development for health educators, including in ethical and safe AI use.

7.1 Introduction

Artificial Intelligence (AI) has a long history, but its impact has only recently come to the fore with the release of publicly accessible online generative AI (GenAI) interfaces such as ChatGPT. The capability of GenAI to produce material in a way that mimics intelligent thought poses many opportunities for health professional educators but also numerous challenges.

In this digital era, health professional curricula need to be re-examined in light of these opportunities and challenges. After a brief introduction to the principles of AI, this chapter will address the core challenges of AI to HPE, divided into three major themes:

1. GenAI has the capability to assist/supplement health professional educators in many aspects of educational curriculum design and delivery. This can be particularly beneficial given that health professional educators are often extremely time-poor [1] and often curricula are dependent upon clinical adjunct staff [2] who have less education-specific training/experience [3] and, thus, less comfort with curricular design than dedicated educational staff.
2. AI has exposed a number of risks and vulnerabilities of current health professional educational methods—particularly in assessment. GenAI has been proven capable of producing answers to essays and exams that pass academic criteria and are extremely difficult to discern from real student work. Given that these assessment forms are regularly used in online health professional educational programs, health professional educators must innovate and adapt their assessments in ways that maintain their integrity in the GenAI era. This may involve using 'AI proof' assessments, such as online viva voces (oral examination), and/or integrating AI more intentionally and transparently into teaching and learning, including assessment, i.e. integrating learning about using AI into the assessment task.
3. As AI is increasingly integrated into healthcare professional practice it is critically important to similarly integrate it into healthcare professional education to prepare graduates with the capabilities to critically use these tools in practice. Therefore, HPE curricula must ensure that AI competencies are being appropriately included into their syllabi.

The chapter will then conclude by providing some roadmaps to assist in guiding institutional and professional responses to AI in digital health education to ensure educators are effectively positioned to constructively utilise this game-changing new technology in their own contexts.

7.2 What Is Artificial Intelligence and how Does it Work?

There are two main forms of AI: Predictive AI and Generative AI. "Predictive AI uses data, such as patient data, to make predictions about future events or trends. Generative AI learns patterns in existing data and generates new data based on those patterns to create original content." [4] While predictive AI has been in use in various forms for many years, it is the significant advances in Generative AI (GenAI) that have proven particularly impactful in health and health education in recent years.

GenAI combines Large Language Models (LLM) with Natural Language Processing (NLP) to create content that mirrors human-generated content. An LLM is a large dataset of human-generated content used to train the model that is then used to statistically predict the most likely sequence of data to generate new content (text, imagery, video content, etc)—hence the term GPT (Generative Pre-Trained Transformer). For example, ChatGPT3.5 (released November 2022) was trained on 17GB of data from 300 billion words [5] whereas ChatGPT4 (released March 2023) was trained on 45GB of data. While the rate of development of GenAI is staggering, it is fundamentally important to realise that GenAI "is not sentient….The operations are based purely on the data used to train the AI models." [6].

GenAI is being integrated into everyday productivity platforms such as Microsoft Office365, Google search, Adobe's creative cloud and Apple Intelligence and accessible directly on devices via various freely available apps. Language translation and writing have been revolutionised by GenAI with LLMs integration into tools such as Grammarly, reducing the barriers for English as second language learners. AI has implications for health professional education, including basic productivity tasks such as note-taking and report writing. It is also impacting the academic integrity of most assessment modes.

It is thus important for HPE educators to be familiar with the opportunities and risks that accompany increased GenAI use and respond appropriately in the design and delivery of educational programming. Each of these will be explored in the following sections of this chapter.

7.3 Opportunities for AI to Aid in the Design and Delivery of HPE Programs

While AI is an actively growing and evolving tool, there are multiple situations where it has already demonstrated its capability to aid in the design and delivery of HPE programs. Here, we describe a number of these key use cases, including some examples of how these can be operationalised.

7.3.1 Improving Educator Productivity

GenAI provides significant opportunities for improving educator productivity by reducing the time taken on administrative and time-consuming written composition tasks. In particular, GenAI can be used to quickly generate the first drafts of a variety of learning designs, such as a curriculum design document, an assessment task outline or assessment marking rubric.

GenAI also has the ability to assist with tasks such as discussion board moderation and assessment feedback, thus potentially freeing educators' capacity for other tasks. However, it should be remembered that AI is producing a response that is templated from other similar responses it has been trained on—therefore, it cannot be guaranteed to produce a response that is appropriate and applicable to the work in question. As such, it is important that when it is used for this purpose, it is done so with full transparency and human oversight.

The following is an example of an AI prompt to generate a first draft of an assessment rubric:

> **Example ChatGPT/Claude3 Sonnet Prompt:** *Act as an expert learning designer in higher education with an extensive knowledge of foundational learning theories and learning design frameworks. Create a Marking Rubric with five quality indicators, each marked out of 20 points of a total of 100 points, for peer review of an academic blog post.*

Practice Point: Prompt Engineering

Effective 'prompt engineering' is the fundamental determinant of the effectiveness of GenAI. It is an iterative process whereby a prompt is developed and refined to appropriately shape the GenAI output to be specific and relevant to the educators' needs. As such, prompt engineering is a skill that all HPE educators, students and health professionals need to develop.

A number of key principles for creating effective AI prompts have been formulated by Meskó [7]:

- Identify the goal of the prompt first

It is important to be completely clear on what you are hoping for the AI to generate to craft the appropriate prompt to do this. Make sure you have articulated this clearly in your own mind before starting to write a prompt.

e.g. The goal may be "The creation of an appropriate assessment to determine a third-year physiotherapy student's understanding of patient management in respiratory intensive care units (RICU) in a wholly online context."

- Be specific

As LLMs are trained on huge datasets, they have the ability to provide outputs that are as generic or specific as the situation needs. In an educational setting, specificity is typically necessary to ensure that the output directly caters to the situation in question.

e.g. Rather than: "Create an assessment rubric for an OSCE examination of the respiratory system?"

Instead, you could ask: "Create an assessment rubric with 5 key criteria for a 10 min OSCE examination of the respiratory system for final year physiotherapy students."

- Provide context

GenAI models are able to tailor their answers to fit different contexts, so these can be built into prompts to help shape the output.

e.g. "The goal is to create an optimal online assessment of third-year physiotherapy student's understanding of patient management in respiratory intensive care units (RICU). With that in mind…."

- Invite role play

An additional way to add context is by inviting the GenAI model to take on a specific 'role' to more accurately represent the situation you are creating the content for.

e.g. "Act as an experienced university physiotherapy lecturer…".

- Varying prompt styles

Different prompt styles will define the structure and format of the GenAI output. Different situations will call for different formats. Vary the prompt style appropriate to meet the relevant need:

e.g.

"What is the best way to…".
"List 3 ways to…."
"Summarise the key ways to…".
"Provide a step-by-step outline of how to…"

- Request examples

Directing the AI to produce an example is an excellent way of ensuring it generates responses that are detailed and concrete.

e.g. "Give specific examples of online activities for assessing third-year physiotherapy student's understanding of patient management in respiratory intensive care units (RICU)."

- Use meta-prompts

GenAI has the ability to respond to meta-prompts. This is an effective way of identifying and learning ways of doing things that an educator would not have independently thought of—including prompt engineering!

e.g. "What prompts would you use to learn the best way to…."

7.3.2 Work-Integrated Learning and Clinical Assessment

GenAI is also being used in work-integrated, clinical education, including in the design and implementation of clinical examinations, such as Objective Structured Clinical Examinations (OSCEs). OSCEs have been used in medical education since the mid 1970s to assess students' clinical skills in history taking, physical examination, clinical reasoning, diagnosis and procedural skills. OSCEs require the administration, design and delivery of complex, validated cases, where a standardized patient (SP) dynamically interacts with trainees, who are observed and receive real-time expert feedback in a controlled environment. This can be resource and time intensive for the educator and stressful for the learner. Although typically conducted face-to-face, the COVID-19 pandemic required experimentation with the use of online teleconference technology to conduct virtual OSCEs. Online resources such as Geeky Medics [8] provide over 1300 OSCE stations across a variety of cases, for students to practice and prepare for their actual examinations. While, as always, there are pros and cons to using GenAI in this context, and it is still in its infancy, AI is transforming the way healthcare professionals can be taught and assessed in this practice-based learning, in face-to-face, virtual, and hybrid environments [9]. A different, but related use of AI is for the creation of 'digital twins' (DT), a virtual representation of a person to predict outcomes and plan treatments based on modelling of multimodal data [10].

The same provisos apply to using GenAI in this context, as indicated above, in relation to privacy, accuracy, safety and integrity. However, GenAI, when overseen by medical educators, can be used in various ways to augment OSCEs, including:

- Determining assessment of clinical skill gaps in general curricular and individual students
- Generating assessment rubrics
- Preparing SPs, with guides, scripts and checklists and using Chatbots, e.g. ChatGPT as 'simulated student', thereby improving exam standardisation, fairness and validity
- Creating novel and tailored OSCE scenarios, stations and cases (See case below)
- Generating mock OSCEs with ChatGPT as a Virtual Standardised Patient (VSP) to help learners prepare, practice and receive feedback in a low-stakes simulation
- Allowing students to practice questioning, history taking and general communication with a virtual standardised patient via ChatGPT [11].

Example: OSCE on clinical examination of suspected gallstones
Example ChatGPT Prompt: Create an OSCE station for the clinical examination of a male patient with suspected gallstones. Include candidate instructions, patient script, examiner instructions and checklist.

7.3.3 Scalable Personalised Learning

The principles of best practice for designing online HPE include personalised learning experiences for individual learners' specific needs, providing timely formative feedback, developing critical reflection and designing assessment that meets specified standards and assesses an individual's progress in understanding and applying concepts. Note, however, that personalised learning requires tracking and data collection through learning analytics, the ethics of which and the necessary consent, data security, ownership and privacy issues must always be considered.

Chickering and Gamson [12] identified seven effective practices that facilitate personalised learning: (1) student-faculty contact, (2) cooperation among students, (3) active learning, (4) prompt feedback, (5) time on task, (6) high expectations, and (7) respect for diverse talents and ways of learning. These are time and resource-intensive and can be achieved with low ratios of students to teachers but become prohibitively expensive at scale. GenAI can provide achievable and cost-effective solutions to scalable personalised learning [13, 14].

AI tutors (ChatBots) can give students immediate personalised feedback based upon information provided by students or their educators on their learning progress [5] and provide suggestions for revision material on a topic or suggestions for the next steps in mastering a topic or concept—acting as a more experienced peer to help students master threshold concepts [15, 16] or dive deeper. AI tutors could learn student preferences for making learning materials more accessible for specific learning needs and (dis)abilities. See Sharples [17] for many other suggestions for AI personalised learning.

MOOCs (Massive Open Online Courses), for example, with little or no individual support, have typically suited the highly self-directed learner [18, 19], but with the integration of GenAI interfaces, there is now the ability to provide participants with personalised immediate support at a scale that is cost-effective and improves participant engagement. Although ChatBots are complex and time consuming to create, open-source development systems such as Rasa [20] and Botpress [21] can assist with designing and training them for use as virtual tutors, and virtual patients such as DeepRaft, a cardiology focused education program for patients and healthcare providers [22].

7.3.4 Scalable, Personalised Support

As all health professional educators know, teaching is not purely about the act of imparting knowledge to a learner. The best teachers are those that can connect with a learner on multiple levels and are able to respond to their human needs. This, in turn, can then prime them for learning success.

Although GenAI cannot feel emotions per se, it can demonstrate a form of emotional intelligence or 'generative AI empathy' whereby it can accurately identify emotions and can respond to them in an emotionally-appropriate way [23, 24].

As such, GenAI has the potential to contribute to the supportive roles that health professional educators regularly provide for their students. This is only an emerging application at this point, but analogous uses have begun to be explored in healthcare provision. This includes utility of AI for behavioural health interventions by using chatbots for digital mental health interventions (DMHI) including cognitive behavioural therapy (CBT) [25, 26]. Other programs such as Hippocratic AI [27] use LLMs to reduce clinician burden and improve patient engagement, while SayHeart simplifies complex health data and medical jargon into patient-friendly visual content [28]. Translation of these applications to the HPE setting is a logical and likely next step.

7.4 Risks and Vulnerabilities that AI Poses to Health Professional Educational Methods

The impact of GenAI on HPE is seen in the challenge to the integrity of traditional assessment designs that have been reliant upon approaches such as essays and exams that are particularly vulnerable to the use of GenAI. How do educators ensure that students have understood and can apply critical concepts rather than simply utilising GenAI to produce assessment artefacts in response to simple prompts without demonstrating acquired competence or developing the appropriate critical thinking skills? Particularly when these skills remain clinically important. A reliance upon AI for diagnostic analysis of patient data without the ability to critically evaluate the validity of the results would be a significant source of clinical risk.

7.4.1 Assessment Integrity

Student submission of assessment tasks that have been produced by GenAI without acknowledgement or critical evaluation of the results is an academic integrity issue similar to plagiarism and is typically subject to the same academic integrity processes.

Although one of the simplest methods to deter GenAI use is through systematic detection methods (and resultant disciplinary processes), this has inherent problems of its own. The rapidly moving pace of AI means that detection algorithms are at constant risk of being unpaced by GenAI technology and, furthermore, the fact that GenAI is trained from real data means that detection systems can never say with 100% certainty that a response was not written by a learner.

Therefore, alternative methods of risk mitigation are necessary, including reworking of assessments to be in formats that are less vulnerable to GenAI. This may include the use of vivas, invigilated examinations, locked-down computer software and limited internet connectivity, the inclusion of AI usage declaration statements, or the purposeful integration of the use of GenAI in the assessment process.

We explore institutional responses to assessment integrity further in Sect. 7.6.

Practice Point: Theoretical Foundations for Optimal AI Assessment Design
Chapter 1 explores core educational theories that can be applied to online education. In this section we explore the application of these theories to AI assessment design and briefly introduce some theoretical foundations not mentioned in Sect. 1.8 that may be useful in guiding the integration of AI in the design of learning and assessment in healthcare professional education.

Cognitive Load Theory (CLT—sect. 1.9.1) focuses on the process of memory retention of information. However, tools such as GenAI can remove some of this load by providing just-in-time access to information and increasing student and practitioner productivity for basic repetitive tasks. This leaves more capacity for students and practitioners to exercise critical judgement and develop creative solutions to problems. Embedding the use of GenAI in creating first drafts of assessments or generating initial concepts for further development is one way to reduce cognitive load.

From a social constructivist perspective (Sect. 1.9.3–1.9.4), AI can be integrated into learning activities and assessment design as a more experienced peer (Context-specific trained ChatBots, for example) to extend learners' zone of proximal development (ZPD) beyond what they could learn on their own [29].

Activity Theory (AT) builds upon social learning theory (Sect. 1.9.4) and provides an analytical framework for identifying the contradictions and strengths in a system that hinder or support the use of technology as a mediating tool to achieve specific learning outcomes [30–34]. For example, institutional policy can be either an enabler (principles-based approach) of the integration of AI in teaching and learning or a blocker (detection-based approaches).

Heutagogy [35–38] takes Andragogy (Sect. 1.9.7) towards Transformative Learning (Sect. 1.9.9), where the focus is on designing learning to enable learner agency and self-determined learning through building students' capacity to navigate the unknown. This relates to building students' capacity for critical thinking and diagnosis in healthcare.

7.4.2 Loss of Critical Graduate Capabilities

As GenAI becomes increasingly accepted and utilised by educators and learners alike, it can be used to remove barriers to the learning process. For instance, GenAI can reduce the language barrier for English as a second language learners by automatically translating text into their native language. AI-powered grammar correction tools such as Grammarly are now part of the toolkit for academic writing. However, the potential for over-reliance on GenAI in this setting is also possible and may create a scenario where learners are no longer able to demonstrate context-appropriate grammatical skills that would be expected in their professional roles.

Therefore, 'hidden curricula' elements, (i.e. elements of learning that are assumed to be acquired (or proven) as part of the normal learning process) may need to be more explicitly considered in the GenAI era, and tasks to ensure these competencies have been achieved may need to be intentionally built into assessment methodology.

7.4.3 Bias

A fundamental issue in the use of GenAI is the explicit and implicit bias introduced through the limitations of the training sources informing these LLMs [39]. AI is trained using available data and the data available on the internet is inherently male and Western first-world dominated. Thus, the bias of the source material will bias the training and therefore the outputs of GenAI, negatively impacting minority and under-represented groups. This can dramatically amplify systemic, historical biases in medicine and healthcare, such as the predominant use of males for medical research or underdiagnosis or misdiagnosis of certain conditions based on gender stereotypes.

7.4.4 Data Integrity and Trust

Another challenge with GenAI is knowing what we can trust, as seeing (or hearing) is no longer believing. GenAI can be used intentionally by humans to deceive, i.e. create 'deep fakes', or it can 'unintentionally' create its own 'hallucinations'. The implications of this are particularly serious in medicine and healthcare. GenAI models are trained to produce 'natural' (human-like) outputs as a primary design objective through generative pre-trained transformers that are basically large predictive statistical models using disaggregated data such that every prompt-based output will be different. In other words, their prime directive is not to be correct. In fact, GenAI models have no capacity to authenticate the validity of their outputs except through a training feedback loop with human trainers. Hence, GenAI can produce errors and incorrect information or outputs that are labelled 'hallucinations' but are fundamentally, simply incorrect outputs. This includes citing references that do not actually exist. Add to this the risk of data obtained without consent, consideration of IP/copyright, or even just correct 'labelling' and the need for a method of warranting the accuracy, authenticity and legality of using data becomes apparent. Indeed, the lack of 'labelling' of medical images is possibly one of medical AI's biggest challenges [40].

7.4.5 The Digital Divide

As with all educational technologies, there is a risk of widening the gap between students from more privileged circumstances and those with less resources and opportunities to use these technologies. Access to technology is determined by the cost of ownership or access to the technology. In the case of GenAI, there is a significant difference in the capabilities of the freely available models and the subscription fee-based state-of-the-art models. Access to computing platforms capable of using GenAI is reduced by the availability of free Apps for mobile devices. However, access to mobile devices capable of AI-on-device will require top-end models with the most powerful processors. The digital divide produced by access to GenAI is compounded by the varied responses to the use of GenAI in education by students, some of whom are reticent to engage with GenAI as an educational tool in case of institutional academic integrity responses. There is emerging evidence [41] of a widening gap between the academic achievement of students with the capacity to appropriately integrate the use of GenAI and those who choose not to.

7.5 Integrating AI Competencies into Curricula

In addition to the potential ways that AI may impact educational processes, it is also important to acknowledge that AI is actively and rapidly becoming incorporated into health professional workflows. Already, AI is being utilised in diagnostic processes, with studies demonstrating that AI has the ability to match or even outdo clinicians in establishing correct diagnoses [42, 43].

AI is also having an emerging role in many other clinical areas, including genomics, drug discovery, clinical trials and dose optimisation, personalised treatment and precision medicine, patient monitoring and mental health care [44, 45]. Given the wide range of applications for AI technology, it is clear that health professionals of the future are going to be utilising AI on a daily basis.

Therefore, the use of common tools, such as ChatGPT (including prompt engineering, as discussed in above in Sect. 7.3.1) could be widely considered to be a core competency for any health professional program and would need to be considered as an addition to current syllabi. More complex AI competencies (for instance, the use of specific diagnostic decision aids, note taking aids, etc.) may also be relevant in specific health professional contexts.

7.6 Roadmap for Institutional Responses to AI

Given that the ramifications of AI are so far-reaching throughout the HPE sector, centralised responses at the institutional level are required to address the major and systematic impacts of this new technology.

Broadly speaking, there are some universal challenges that AI poses that will need to be considered by every institution, even if the specific way they choose to respond to this is different. As such, here we present a basic roadmap for HPE organisations which can then be used to template their individualized responses to AI.

7.6.1 Development of Principles Governing the Use of AI

HPE organisations must begin by creating overriding principles that will shape all internal policies and actions regarding AI. These create a unifying framework that can be referred to as a guide for all downstream decision-making.

A useful prototype for these principles is the five principles on the use of generative AI tools in education, released by the Russell Group of universities in the United Kingdom (UK) [46]. These principles were also expanded upon by the Joint Information Systems Committee (JISC) in the UK, which is a not-for-profit organisation that provides IT services and digital resources in support of further education in the UK [47].

The five principles are:

1. Universities will support students and staff to become AI-literate.
2. Staff should be equipped to support students to use generative AI tools effectively and appropriately in their learning experience.
3. Universities will adapt teaching and assessment to incorporate the ethical use of generative AI and support equal access.
4. Universities will ensure academic rigour and integrity are upheld.
5. Universities will work collaboratively to share best practices as the technology and its application in education evolves.

7.6.2 Copyright, IP and Privacy

Most GenAI models are owned by large private companies whose copyright and intellectual property policies do not necessarily match those of the educational institutions using them. Data sovereignty is an issue—where the data used for training the models or the data uploaded to the models is stored and who has access to this information and data. Training data for GenAI comes from many sources and models are sometimes trained without the necessary permissions to use the data (text, images, video, audio, etc) from the copyright owners. For HPE organisations, this may mean that educators are uploading copyright-restricted materials, including institutionally owned teaching resources or student data or information that should not be shared in the public domain. To address this, institutions can develop their own GenAI models as noted above or utilise private password-protected gateways to GenAI models that have specific restrictions placed upon data storage, privacy and training datasets.

7.6.3 Mitigating Bias

In the process of establishing organisation specific AIs, or organisation-specific AI subsets, limitations can be placed on GenAI models to try and mitigate this bias or reduce the malicious use of GenAI to produce politically biased or other harmful fake outputs.

Where an institution has trained an AI specifically upon its own datasets, the risk of bias is reduced, assuming the datasets are representative of the cohort in question, thereby mitigating against risks of trust, validation, privacy and IP/copyright breaches.

7.6.4 Encouraging/Ensuring Widespread AI Literacy

Given the range of opportunities and risks associated with the use of GenAI in higher education, there is a critical need for raising the awareness of both students and staff of the implications of these. The direct impact upon academic integrity, the unreliability of detection of the use of GenAI and the fundamental principles of when and how to critically engage with GenAI in teaching and learning require new strategies for staff professional development and student digital literacy development. Ignoring the issues and leaving a response up to individuals is not an option, given the push by governmental policies.

7.6.5 Detection

The two fundamental approaches to ensuring academic integrity in assessment have been assuring the integrity of assessment through invigilation or detection. Detection tools such as Turnitin have been widely institutionalised for detecting plagiarism in assessments submitted by students and are increasingly also used by academic publishers to detect plagiarism in academic papers submitted to journals and books. However, early attempts at using detection tools to identify the unacceptable or undeclared use of GenAI in writing have produced both false positives and false negatives. As the level of sophistication of GenAI models rapidly increases, the lag between the capabilities of these tools and the detection of their use is problematic. The nature of GPTs behind GenAI models means that data used in their training or uploaded through prompts is disaggregated from the source material, and no two prompt results will be the same, making detection very difficult. To mitigate the issues with unreliable detection of the inappropriate use of GenAI tools, institutions and publishers are introducing declaration statements for students or academics to expressly acknowledge how they may have used GenAI in any academic writing as an ethical approach to the issue.

7.6.6 Modelling the Professional Use of AI

As AI and GenAI continues to be integrated into the fundamental workflows of students, healthcare educators need professional development in order to develop praxis that embeds the critical and professional use of these tools and are also responsible for modelling the professional and appropriate use of these tools to their students. The development of critical judgement in when and how to use these tools is essential for students and academics [48].

Integrating existing, validated clinical AI and GenAI applications into education and training programs is one way to model and critically appraise their appropriate use. This is obviously contingent upon privacy, copyright, IP and other access issues for teaching institutions in relation to such software. The following two examples suggest how existing clinical AI augmented programs might be used for education purposes. The first is in medical imaging, which, as noted earlier is leading the way in medical AI use. The second is a clinical pilot of an AI-based hospital sepsis prediction system.

Example 1: Open-Source Software for Medical Imaging AI
Microsoft's Project InnerEye is an open-source software (OSS), designed for deep learning research and available free via the Massachusetts Institute of Technology (MIT) License for the global medical imaging community [49]. It is intended for clinicians such as radiologists and organisations to build, adapt and deploy their own models for analysing 3D medical images, but it could also be used for radiologist training purposes. One of its most prominent projects is OSAIRIS, a cloud-based software developed by the University of Cambridge and Cambridge University Hospitals National Health Service (NHS) Foundation [50]. It uses AI to complete time-consuming 3D segmentation of normal from cancerous tissues during radiotherapy planning of head and neck, and prostate cancers, allowing doctors to focus on treatment planning and reduce patient waiting times.

In an educational context, a version of this program, trained with approved 'de-identified' images, could be used by students in conjunction with traditional segmentation methods to critically compare these approaches and learn when and how AI might be best used in a professional clinical context.

Example 2: Hospital Sepsis Prediction
eHealth NSW (New South Wales, Australia) have developed an AI-based prediction system that draws upon electronic medical record (eMR) data to calculate a patient's risk of developing sepsis (approximately 5%–7% of patient presentations, with a 20% risk of death) in emergency departments (ED). If successful, this is intended to replace paper-based, manual-calculation prediction systems, which historically often miss true positives and generate higher false positives. The AI program uses three different models, monitored by Amazon SageMaker, for greater accuracy across a range of patients. The sepsis risk prediction is presented to clinicians via a Tableau Dashboard to inform potential earlier interventions [51]. In an educational context, institutional access to this eHealth NSW program, or a specific training version thereof with deidentified or simulated patient data, would allow medical students and trainee nurses to practice using this predictive technology in conjunction with paper-based approaches. This would allow them to critically compare and contrast these approaches and develop insight into using such AI-based systems.

7.7 Roadmap for Educators' Individual Professional Development in AI

UNESCO's 2023 report [5] suggests a range of options for critically integrating GenAI into assessment, teaching and learning activities. Many of these require a fundamental shift in the role of the educator from being the deliverer of content knowledge to being the designer of authentic learning experiences. This requires professional development for educators—we explore this in the following sections of this chapter.

7.7.1 *Technical Pedagogical and Content Knowledge*

The Technical Pedagogical and Content Knowledge (TPACK) framework [52] **(introduced in chap. 2)** articulates three fundamental capability areas for educators in the age of digital learning. The framework applies broadly to the use of any digital tools and can be a useful framework for identifying the professional education capabilities needed in response to the use of GenAI in teaching and learning. GenAI impacts all three areas of educator knowledge: technical knowledge of the fundamentals of how GenAI works, how to utilise it in teaching and learning, and the specific risks and opportunities of the use of GenAI in a specific discipline context. Thus, educators should seek out professional development that specifically upskills them in the use of GenAI across these three domains and is relevant to their HPE context (see Sect. 7.7.3 for some specific resources).

7.7.2 Rethinking the Role of the Educator

GenAI requires a fundamental shift in the role of the educator from being the deliverer of content knowledge to being the designer of authentic learning experiences. This fundamental shift is in tension with the TPACK framework, where the focus is clearly upon content knowledge and does not highlight the need to rethink the educator's role as a gatekeeper of content knowledge. This is where we must draw upon a wider set of theoretical foundations as identified in sect. 7.7.3, such as facilitating self-determined learning and building students' capacity to navigate the unknown as highlighted by Heutagogy [36, 38, 53–55] and Rhizomatic learning, [56, 57] where the role of the educator shifts to becoming a designer of learning experiences as triggering events to guide students exploration of appropriate areas of knowledge and critical thinking.

7.7.3 AI Implementation Frameworks

As part of the Educational Sector-wide response to the emergence of AI, a number of implementation frameworks have begun to be published as learning design resources [5, 14, 58–61]. These can serve as further reading on how to effectively integrate AI into health professional education.

- The Deloitte report "From code to cure, how Generative AI can reshape the health frontier: Unlocking new levels of efficiency, effectiveness, and innovation" [59] provides practical advice for the health sector.
- The IDEE framework [14] is a relatively simple theoretical framework that has four steps in using GenAI in education: **I**dentify the desired outcomes, **D**etermine the appropriate level of automation, **E**nsure ethical considerations, and **E**valuate the effectiveness.
- Crawford et al., [60] offer suggestions for using AI in academic publishing processes.
- Liu and Bridgeman [58] expand upon the University of Sydney Two-Lane approach to AI in education.
- UNESCO offers practical advice in a quick start guide [5] building upon the work of Sharples examples of how AI could be implemented in teaching and learning.
- The PAIR framework for using GenAI in education is similar to the IDEE framework, identifying four steps: **P**roblem, **A**I, **I**nteraction, **R**eflection [61].

7.8 Considering the Ethics of AI in Healthcare

An essential element of online HPE is encouraging learners to reflect critically upon key ethical issues concerning AI in medicine and healthcare. These include issues relating to patient safety, algorithmic fairness and biases, informed consent for the use of personal data and health records, and data security, ownership, privacy and confidentiality [62]. Helpfully, many of these complex ethical considerations apply not only to healthcare but to online teaching and learning practice, where the student can substitute for the patient and the teacher for the HCP. There is the opportunity, therefore, to use online HPE to model ethical best practice use of AI.

Online HPE should foster reflexive practitioners who are always considering how AI (in both their clinical practice and their education) affects their own professional practices, thinking processes and identities. 'Big' questions should be considered by both HPE teachers and learners, such as How does AI change the nature of healthcare and my role in it? What is the patient experience of AI-augmented healthcare? How does AI impact my 'cognitive apprenticeship' and the way I think and clinically reason? How much autonomy should AI have, and indeed, should AI have its own rights?

GenAI requires human oversight and critical evaluation of the results [60, 63, 64]. A tendency of an Actor-Network Theory approach (See sect. 1.8.8) to technology reinforces the anthropomorphism of GenAI, assigning the same agency to GenAI as to humans rather than focusing upon developing student reflexivity. A better approach may be to conceptualise human-AI interaction as a co-creation process such as Activity Theory [33, 34, 65] that conceptualises tools as mediators of learning rather than independent actors.

As we move from a phase of suspicion and detection to one of transparency, open collaboration, co-creation between teachers and learners, AI will undoubtedly be a key tool that can facilitate this transition, but it must be managed sensibly and proactively to ensure its potential is used in ways that are ultimately beneficial for HPE rather than detrimental.

7.9 Tips and Tricks

- When thinking about AI
    - Take a positive, proactive mindset to the opportunities of the technology. Like the internet and smartphones, the use of AI will only increase in the coming years, so becoming familiar is not something that can be avoided.
    - Embrace an attitude of collaboration and transparency between teachers and learners who can both benefit from its use rather than an attitude of need for detection and enforcement.
    - Learn from example—GenAI interfaces can be complex, and their prompting syntaxes are complex. Worked examples (including those in this chapter, and

others published online) can provide templates that can fast-track an individual to produce the type of output they need in an HPE setting.

- When familiarising oneself with AI interfaces
  - Take the time to actively explore and experiment with AI interfaces as they appear. While this appears to be a confronting new technique, the time invested will pay dividends due to the high productivity yields of GenAI interfaces.
  - Don't limit yourself to a single AI interface (e.g. ChatGPT). Many different models are publicly available online for different academic purposes and have different strengths and weaknesses.
- When designing assessments
  - Static assessments, which are focused around a single, refined final output (such as essays), are the types of assessments that are most vulnerable to AI replication. As such, their utility is likely to decrease in time.
  - Real-time assessments including OSCEs, viva voce exams, oral presentations and practical tasks are all tasks that are not easily replicated by AI.
  - Consider utilising methods that involve active reflection, leverage personal experiences (i.e. that an AI model would not know of) and methods that require the learner to document the meta-cognitive processes that led to an outcome. Again, these are not easily replicated by AI.

7.10 Conclusion

Artificial Intelligence has a major role to play in the education of future health professionals. It can and will be utilised to assist in the design and delivery of education and should be embraced by health professional educators to enhance teaching programs. AI will undoubtedly influence how we think about healthcare from now on and, therefore, must be part of HPE curricula. Given its emergent and hyper-evolving nature, however, it is impossible ever to be fully up to date with AI in HPE, healthcare or anywhere. Therefore, we emphasise great importance in preparing health professionals to think critically about AI and to consider its broader ethical implications, including for their professional roles and identities, not just learning how to use specific applications. Online HPE is well placed to use AI in its teaching and learning and, in so doing, model and foster informed decision-making about current and emerging clinical AI applications and, most importantly, what data can be trusted. In other words, online HPE must now embrace learning with, from and about AI.

References

1. Goldie J, et al. The influence of structural and institutional change on teaching and culture in clinical settings: an exploratory study. Med Teach. 2015;37(2):189–95.
2. Dutt S, Phelps M, Scott KM. Curricular change and delivery promotes teacher development and engagement. High Educ Res Dev. 2020;39(7):1425–39.
3. Riesenberg LA, Little BW, Wright V. Nonphysician medical educators: a literature review and job description resource. Acad Med. 2009;84(8):1078–88.
4. Harrington L. Comparison of generative artificial intelligence and predictive artificial intelligence. AACN Adv Crit Care. 2024;35(2):93–6.
5. Sabzalieva E, Valentini A ChatGPT and artificial intelligence in higher education: quick start guide. UNESCO International Institute for Higher Education in Latin America and the Caribbean (IESALC). 2023. p. 14
6. Educause Review. 7 Things you should know about generative AI. Educ Rev. 2023;2023
7. Meskó B. Prompt engineering as an important emerging skill for medical professionals: tutorial. J Med Internet Res. 2023;25:e50638.
8. Potter L. *OSCE stations*. In: *Geeky medics*; 2022.
9. Soong TK, Ho CM. Artificial intelligence in medical OSCEs: reflections and future developments. Adv Med Educ Pract. 2021;12:167–73.
10. Katsoulakis E, et al. Digital twins for health: a scoping review. npj Digital Medicine. 2024;7(1):77.
11. Misra SM, Suresh S. Artificial intelligence and objective structured clinical examinations: using ChatGPT to revolutionize clinical skills assessment in medical education. J Med Educat Curri Develop. 2024;11:23821205241263475.
12. Chickering AW, Gamson ZF. Seven principles for good practice in undergraduate education. AAHE Bull. 1987;3:7.
13. Wu R, Yu Z. Do AI chatbots improve students learning outcomes? Evidence from a meta-analysis. Br J Educ Technol. 2024;55(1):10–33.
14. Su J, Yang W. Unlocking the power of ChatGPT: a framework for applying generative AI in education. ECNU Rev Educ. 2023;6(3):355–66.
15. Anderson T. Theories with learning with emerging technologies. In: Veletsianos G, editor. Emergence and innovation in digital learning: foundations and applications. Canada: Athabasca University Press; 2016. p. 35–50.
16. Land R, et al. Threshold concepts and troublesome knowledge (3)*: implications for course design and evaluation. In: Rust C, editor. Improving student learning diversity and inclusivity. Oxford: Oxford Centre for Staff and Learning Development; 2005. p. 53–64.
17. Sharples M. Towards social generative AI for education: theory, practices and ethics. Learn: Res Pract. 2023;9(2):159–67.
18. Stacey P. Pedagogy of MOOCs. Int J Innov Qual Learn. 2014;2(3) (Special Issue on Quality in Massive Open Online Courses):112–5.
19. Koller D, et al. Retention and intention in massive open online courses: in depth. EDUCAUSE Rev Online. 2013;
20. RASA AI. Available from: https://rasa.com/
21. BotPress AI. Available from: https://botpress.com/
22. DeepDraft AI. Available from: https://deepraft.com/
23. Ayers JW, et al. Comparing physician and artificial intelligence chatbot responses to patient questions posted to a public social media forum. JAMA Intern Med. 2023;183(6):589–96.
24. Inzlicht M, et al. In praise of empathic AI. Trends Cogn Sci. 2023;
25. Egan SJ, et al. A pilot study of the perceptions and acceptability of guidance using artificial intelligence in internet cognitive behaviour therapy for perfectionism in young people. Internet Interv. 2024;35:100711.
26. Al-Wahedi M, et al. Automation of electronic cognitive Behavioural therapy (automated-eCBT) in adapting psychotherapy in a clinical context: a review. Psychology. 2024;15(9):1474–503.

27. Hippocratic AI. Available from: https://www.hippocraticai.com/
28. SayHeart AI. Available from: https://sayheart.ai/
29. Head G, Dakers J. Verillon's trio and Wenger's community: learning in technology education. Int J Technol Des Educ. 2005;15:33–46.
30. Kwong C-YC, Churchill D. Applying the activity theory framework to analyse the use of ePortfolios in an international baccalaureate middle years Programme sciences classroom: a longitudinal multiple-case study. Comput Educ. 2023;200:104792.
31. Schmidt M, Tawfik A. Activity theory as a lens for developing and applying personas and scenarios in learning experience design. 2022;11: p. 13
32. Kamanga R, Alexander PM. Contradictions and strengths in activity systems: enhancing insights into human activity in IS adoption research. Elec J Info Syst Dev Countries. 2021;87(1):e12149.
33. Engeström Y. Expansive learning at work: toward an activity theoretical reconceptualization. J Educ Work. 2001;14(1):133–56.
34. Leont'ev AN. Activity, consciouness, and personality. Englewood Cliffs: Prentice Hall; 1978.
35. Lynch M, et al. A heutagogical approach for the assessment of internet communication technology (ICT) assignments in higher education. Int J Educ Technol High Educ. 2021;18(1):55.
36. Hase S, Blaschke LM, editors. Unleashing the power of learner agency. EdTech Books; 2021.
37. Blaschke LM, Hase S. Heutagogy and digital media networks: setting students on the path to lifelong learning. Pacific J Technol Enhanc Learn. 2019;1(1):1–14.
38. Hase S, Kenyon C. Heutagogy: a child of complexity theory. Complicity: Int J Comp Edu. 2007;4(1):111–8.
39. IBM Data and AI Team. Shedding light on AI bias with real world examples. 2023 [cited 2024 27 July]; Available from: https://www.ibm.com/blog/shedding-light-on-ai-bias-with-real-world-examples/
40. Morales S, Engan K, Naranjo V. Artificial intelligence in computational pathology–challenges and future directions. Digit Signal Process. 2021;119:103196.
41. Lodge J. AI in the wild: how students are using generative AI in their learning. Pacific J Technol Enhanc Learn. 2024;6(1):1.
42. Ghaffar Nia N, Kaplanoglu E, Nasab A. Evaluation of artificial intelligence techniques in disease diagnosis and prediction. Discov Artif Intell. 2023;3(1):5.
43. Salinas MP, et al. A systematic review and meta-analysis of artificial intelligence versus clinicians for skin cancer diagnosis. npj Digital Med. 2024;7(1):125.
44. Alowais SA, et al. Revolutionizing healthcare: the role of artificial intelligence in clinical practice. BMC Medical Education. 2023;23(1):689.
45. Iqbal J, et al. Reimagining healthcare: unleashing the power of artificial intelligence in medicine. Cureus. 2023;15(9)
46. Russell Group. Russell Group principles on the use of generative AI tools in education. 2023 4 July [cited 2024 14 August]; Available from: https://russellgroup.ac.uk/media/6137/rg_ai_principles-final.pdf
47. JISC. Principles for the use of AI in FE colleges. 2023 [cited 2024 14 August]; Available from: https://www.jisc.ac.uk/further-education-and-skills/principles-for-the-use-of-ai-in-fe-colleges
48. Mollick E, Mollick E. Co-intelligence. Random House UK. 2024
49. Microsoft Health Futures. Project InnerEye—Democratizing Medical Imaging AI. 2024; [cited 2024 28 August]; Available from: https://www.microsoft.com/en-us/research/project/medical-image-analysis/
50. Cambridge Enterprise. OSAIRIS: AI cancer imaging tool. 2024;[cited 2024 28 August]; Available from: https://www.enterprise.cam.ac.uk/opportunities/osairis-ai-cancer-imaging-tool/
51. Hendry J. eHealth NSW is using AI to detect sepsis in hospital admissions. itnews 2022, May 25;[cited 2024 28 August]; Available from: https://www.itnews.com.au/news/ehealth-nsw-is-using-ai-to-detect-sepsis-in-hospital-admissions-580419

52. Voogt J, et al. Technological pedagogical content knowledge—a review of the literature. J Comput Assist Learn. 2012;29(2):109–21.
53. Kavashev Z. A bibliometric performance analysis of publication productivity within pedagogy, andragogy, and heutagogy continuum: outcomes of SciVal analytics. E-Learning and Digital Media. 2024;0:20427530241239406.
54. Moore RL. Developing lifelong learning with heutagogy: contexts, critiques, and challenges. Distance Education. 2020;41(3):381–401.
55. Hase S, Kenyon C. *From andragogy to Heutagogy*. ultiBASE Articles. 2001:1–10.
56. Blaschke LM, Bozkurt A, Cormier D. Learner agency and the learner-Centred theories for online networked learning and learning ecologies. In: Hase S, Blaschke LM, editors. Unleashing the power of learner agency. EdTech Books; 2021.
57. Cormier D. Rhizomatic education: community as curriculum. Innovate. 2008;4(5) p. np. Available http://davecormier.com/edblog/2008/06/03/rhizomatic-education-community-as-curriculum/
58. Liu D, Bridgeman A. Rules, access, familiarity, and trust—a practical approach to addressing generative AI in education. In: Teaching@Sydney. University of Sydney; 2024.
59. Deloitte. From code to cure, how Generative AI can reshape the health frontier: unlocking new levels of efficiency, effectiveness, and innovation. 2024; p. 24
60. Crawford J, Allen K-A, Lodge J. Humanising peer review with artificial intelligence: paradox or panacea? J Univ Teach Learn Pract. 2024;21(1)
61. Acar O. Are your students ready for AI? A 4-step framework to prepare learners for a ChatGPT world. Educ Technol. 2023; [cited 2024 29 July]; Available from: https://hbsp.harvard.edu/inspiring-minds/are-your-students-ready-for-ai?
62. Gerke S, Minssen T, Cohen G. Ethical and legal challenges of artificial intelligence-driven healthcare. In: Artificial intelligence in healthcare. Elsevier; 2020. p. 295–336.
63. Pelletier K, et al. EDUCAUSE horizon report teaching and learning edition, in EDUCAUSE horizon report. 2023, Educause
64. Selkrig M, et al. Keeping it human: learning design in the digital age. In: MGSE industry reports. Melbourne, Australia: The University of Melbourne Faculty of Education; 2023. p. 32.
65. Bozalek V, et al. Activity theory, authentic learning and emerging technologies: towards a transformative higher education pedagogy. Routledge; 2014. p. 246.

Chapter 8
Implementing and Leading Online Education Transformation

David Bowser

Abstract This chapter explores the process of leading and implementing digital transformations in educational institutions, particularly in the context of online education. It highlights the key challenges, such as faculty resistance, infrastructure demands, and the necessity for proper faculty training. Additionally, it delves into the strategic role leadership plays in fostering a smooth and effective digital transition. The chapter emphasizes the importance of aligning digital transformation with the institution's objectives, equipping faculty with the necessary skills, and ensuring the ongoing quality of education through robust assessment and evaluation methods. Using case studies and research-backed strategies, the chapter provides practical guidance for leaders navigating the complexities of online education transformation.

Key Points Challenges of Resistance: Overcoming resistance from faculty and students is key to digital learning success, with clear communication and early involvement of stakeholders being crucial.

- Infrastructure and Resources: Institutions must invest in robust infrastructure, ensuring equitable access to technology and continuous updates to digital platforms.
- Faculty Development: Effective digital transformation requires ongoing faculty training and support tailored to individual needs and teaching styles.
- Strategic Leadership: Successful leadership involves setting clear goals, appointing dedicated teams, and maintaining open communication with all stakeholders.
- Assessment and Evaluation: Regular assessments and feedback loops are necessary to ensure the quality of digital learning and to refine strategies continuously.
- Case Studies: Three practical examples from educational institutions illustrate how leadership, strategic planning, and stakeholder engagement are crucial to achieving digital transformation.

D. Bowser (✉)
Curio Group, Melbourne, VIC, Australia
e-mail: david.bowser@curiogroup.com

© The Author(s), under exclusive license to Springer Nature Switzerland AG 2025
D. L. Kok et al. (eds.), *Best Practices in Online Education*, IAMSE Manuals,
https://doi.org/10.1007/978-3-031-90349-6_8

8.1 Introduction

Leading an online education transformation is an exciting, and privileged, position to be in. The move to an online environment is one of the most significant paradigm changes that may occur in any learning program, with widespread ramifications for pedagogy, student learning and program logistics—as has already been discussed in previous chapters. With global trends shifting rapidly, particularly underlined by recent events like the COVID-19 pandemic, it is imperative for educational institutions to be able to adapt and fully embrace the potential of online education. This move is not just a temporary adjustment but a key step towards a more inclusive, adaptable, and forward-thinking educational landscape. (Further details on the broader context in which online education occurs are discussed in Chap. 3.).

In this chapter we will explore the practicalities of leading an online transformation and provide advice on how to effectively lead such a complex process. This begins with a discussion of the significant challenges one must be aware of that can impede the change process. The reluctance to embrace change, the necessity for sufficient infrastructure, and the imperative of equipping faculty with the necessary skills are prominent challenges. These challenges are balanced by the opportunities presented by digital learning, such as enhanced accessibility, tailored learning experiences, and improved student engagement.

Our focus is on strategic leadership as a critical factor in successful digital transformation. Aligning this shift with organisational objectives, investing in solid infrastructure, and supporting faculty are crucial. Additionally, we highlight the importance of maintaining high-quality learning experiences, emphasising effective assessment and evaluation methods in digital formats.

Of course, no two transformations will be the same. They vary in their contexts, their size, the drivers and resourcing. As such, there is no exact set recipe for success. However, there are several core considerations and universal steps that must be traversed as part of the process. This chapter outlines the key elements to helping formulate a comprehensive, individualized implementation strategy. We propose a way forward that not only addresses immediate needs for transitioning to digital platforms but also considers the long-term impact on students, educators, and the educational system at large. This transformation, we argue, is about re-envisioning the future of learning, not merely adopting new technologies.

8.2 Challenges

One of the significant challenges in digital learning transformation is resistance from faculty, staff, and students who favour traditional teaching methods. For instance, at universities where lecturers have long relied on face-to-face interactions and established curricula, the introduction of a digital platform might be met with scepticism from faculty concerned about the impersonal nature of online teaching or anxious about mastering new technologies. Similarly, students accustomed to on-campus experiences may initially resist virtual classrooms.

To overcome this resistance, it is essential to demonstrate the tangible benefits of digital learning. Benefits include the flexibility to access materials anytime, the ability to use interactive multimedia for complex subjects, and opportunities for collaboration across geographical boundaries. Research supports these strategies, as shown in studies [1, 2] which emphasise the importance of addressing concerns and involving stakeholders early in the process to gain their buy-in. After initial reluctance, faculty might discover that digital tools allow for more personalised feedback, while students might find that online forums provide a space for deeper discussion. This realisation helps transform the shift to digital learning from a forced march into a collective journey.

Universities must invest in robust infrastructure to support their digital learning initiatives. This involves ensuring that all students and faculty have access to adequate hardware, such as computers or tablets, essential for participating in online classes and accessing course materials. Additionally, institutions must maintain up-to-date software, including learning management systems and various educational tools, which need regular updates to incorporate the latest features and security measures. This infrastructure acts as the backbone of digital education, supporting a seamless transition from traditional to digital learning environments. Porter and Graham [3] identified that sufficient infrastructure, technological support, and pedagogical support are crucial for faculty adoption of blended learning.

Proper training and support for faculty and staff are paramount for the effective adoption of digital learning tools. Designing and implementing comprehensive training programs that introduce the necessary technical skills and pedagogical approaches suited for digital education is crucial. Liu et al. [1] highlight that tailored training and continuous support are vital for ensuring faculty confidence and competence in delivering quality education through digital mediums. These programs must be scalable to accommodate limited resources and provide ongoing support, including troubleshooting and pedagogical advice, to help staff continuously refine their approach to digital teaching. King and Boyatt [4] also emphasize the importance of varied staff development programs and opportunities for sharing practices among colleagues to support e-learning adoption.

Maintaining educational quality during the shift to digital learning is vital. Universities must ensure that digital courses are well-designed to meet learning objectives effectively. This involves creating engaging and interactive content, designing assessments that accurately measure student understanding, and employing varied delivery methods to cater to different learning styles. Continuous quality assurance processes are necessary to evaluate and improve the digital learning experience, ensuring it remains at par with, if not superior to, traditional learning modalities. Yan and Lindner [5] found that factors such as professional area, level of education, and teaching experience significantly influence faculty adoption behaviour in web-based distance education, highlighting the need for tailored approaches based on these variables.

By addressing these challenges strategically and leveraging insights from relevant studies, institutions can facilitate a smoother transition to digital learning, fostering a more adaptable and inclusive educational environment.

8.3 Implementing digital learning transformations

Earlier in this chapter, we outlined the challenges and opportunities that transforming your learning for digital delivery provides. In this section, we provide an outline of what you need to do in your 6–12-month plan of transformation.

We cover the following major points with case studies and examples:

1. Leadership and vision
2. Develop a plan for the transformation
3. Infrastructure and resources
4. Faculty development and training
5. Assessment and evaluation

8.3.1 Strategic Leadership and Vision

Leading a successful digital transformation in learning requires a confluence of strong leadership, strategic planning, and clear communication. At the heart of this shift is the establishment of a vision that aligns with the educational institution's mission and the practical steps necessary to realize it. This begins with appointing a dedicated leadership team, setting clear and attainable goals, and engaging all stakeholders in the vision for change. The introduction of these elements sets the stage for a university to not only adopt digital learning technologies but to do so in a way that enhances educational outcomes and equips students for the future.

You should take the following steps:

- **Appoint a leadership team**: Identify and empower individuals or teams with a clear mandate to spearhead digital initiatives. These leaders should be advocates for change, with a blend of strategy, educational insight and technological acumen.
- **Define clear goals**: Set specific, measurable, achievable, relevant, and time-bound (SMART) objectives that resonate with the broader educational outcomes of the university.
- **Communicate the vision**: Develop a communication plan that articulates the benefits and expected outcomes of digital transformation to all stakeholders, including faculty, staff, students, and possibly even parents and alumni.
- **Stakeholders buy-in**: Use town halls, workshops, and feedback sessions to engage stakeholders, fostering a sense of ownership and addressing concerns proactively.

- **Monitor and adapt**: Establish a feedback loop to monitor progress towards goals, using data to make informed decisions and adapting the strategy as needed.

8.3.1.1 Case Study: University Medical School

A leading university medical school embarked on a digital transformation to enhance educational outcomes and prepare medical students for the future. The initiative aimed to leverage online learning technologies to create a more inclusive, adaptable, and forward-thinking learning environment. An experienced educator with a strong background in technology integration was appointed as the team leader including experts in educational technology, curriculum development, and IT infrastructure to spearhead the initiatives.

The team set specific, measurable, achievable, relevant, and time-bound (SMART) objectives, including implementing a sub-branch of a new Learning Management System within six months, training all faculty members in online teaching tools within a year, increasing student engagement through interactive digital content by 50% in the next academic year, and enhancing online accessibility for remote and international students. A robust communication plan ensured everyone within the school understood the vision, using emails, newsletters, and town hall meetings to share updates. Workshops and training sessions helped faculty and staff grasp their roles in this transformation.

Stakeholder engagement was crucial. The team organised town halls, workshops, and feedback sessions to allow faculty, staff, students, employers and even alumni to voice concerns and offer suggestions, fostering a sense of ownership and collaboration. A feedback loop was established to monitor progress towards goals, allowing the team to make informed decisions and adapt strategies as needed. For instance, when initial feedback showed some faculty struggled with the new LMS experience, additional training and one-on-one support was provided.

This transformation demonstrates the power of strong leadership, strategic planning, and clear communication. By appointing a dedicated leadership team, setting clear goals, engaging stakeholders, and continuously monitoring progress, the university successfully navigated this transformative journey. As a result, the institution not only adopted digital learning technologies but also significantly enhanced its educational outcomes, preparing students for the future of medicine.

8.3.2 *Planning for Digital Transformation*

Developing a project plan for digital transformation involves establishing clear objectives and milestones that align with the broader educational goals. It also requires a comprehensive approach, coordinating between technology, pedagogy, and organizational change management to ensure a seamless integration into the existing educational framework.

In our experience with many education providers, we take the following approach:

1. **Define project scope**: Identify and document specific areas that digital transformation will impact, such as course delivery, student services, or administrative operations. This clarity will prevent scope creep and keep the project focused.
2. **Assemble a cross-functional team**: Bring together a diverse team with members from academics, IT, administration, and student representatives. This ensures that the project benefits from a variety of perspectives and expertise.
3. **Develop a transformation roadmap**: Create a phased plan that starts with quick wins to build momentum and outlines subsequent phases with clear deadlines. This plan will serve as a guide for the project's lifecycle. (See Table 8.1)
4. **Allocate resources**: Determine the budget, technology, equipment, and personnel necessary for each stage of the project. Securing these resources upfront can prevent bottlenecks later.
5. **Risk management**: Conduct a thorough risk assessment to identify potential obstacles and develop strategies for risk mitigation. This proactive approach helps in maintaining project stability.
6. **Monitor progress**: Use project management tools to track progress against the roadmap. Regular monitoring helps in identifying deviations early and making necessary adjustments.
7. **Communicate regularly**: Establish a communication plan that addresses how updates are to be communicated to stakeholders. Regular and clear communication helps in managing expectations and ensuring buy-in.

8.3.3 Infrastructure and Resources Support

To effectively support digital learning, you should focus on creating a robust and scalable IT infrastructure that prioritises educational needs. This means ensuring high-speed internet connectivity to facilitate seamless access to learning management systems, sufficient bandwidth to accommodate resource-intensive applications, and the availability of relevant digital tools and technologies that enhance interactive learning. Continuous updates and maintenance of these systems are essential to harness the full potential of digital learning and improve educational outcomes.

Here are some steps you should consider:

1. **Learning-centric IT systems**: Upgrade IT systems specifically to support interactive and multimedia content delivery, crucial for modern learning environments.
2. **Reliable internet for learning platforms**: Ensure campus-wide, high-speed internet that can support learning management systems and virtual classroom software without interruptions.

8 Implementing and Leading Online Education Transformation

Table 8.1 Example of a transformation roadmap

Phase	Phase 1: Planning and leadership (Months 1–2)	Phase 2: Infrastructure setup and pilot Testing (Months 3–6)	Phase 3: Faculty training and development (Months 4–8)	Phase 4: Full implementation and Rollout (Months 6–10)	Phase 5: Assessment, evaluation, and continuous improvement (Months 10–12 and beyond)
Objectives	• Establish leadership and project governance. • Define vision, goals, and success metrics.	• Build the digital infrastructure. • Conduct pilot programs for early feedback.	• Equip faculty with digital teaching skills. • Provide continuous support and training.	• Scale digital learning to full implementation. • Ensure continuous monitoring and improvement.	• Measure outcomes and success of the transformation. • Adapt strategies based on data and feedback.
Activities	• Appoint leadership team • Conduct stakeholder workshops • Define goals • Develop project plan • Conduct needs assessment.	• Upgrade IT infrastructure • Provide digital tools • Pilot select courses • Collect feedback.	• Develop faculty development programs • Offer workshops • Establish technical support • Encourage peer learning.	• Roll out digital learning across all courses • Monitor transition • Gather performance metrics • Address issues.	• Conduct formal assessments • Use learning analytics • Refine tools and methods • Develop long-term strategy.
Milestones	• Leadership team appointed • Vision and goals defined • Project plan approved.	• Infrastructure upgrades completed • Pilot programs launched • Feedback collected.	• Faculty development programs implemented • Majority of faculty trained • Technical support operational.	• Full rollout of digital learning, progress reports provided • Continuous feedback loops established.	• Assessment reports completed • Continuous improvement strategies implemented • Long-term strategy adopted.

3. **Bandwidth for educational tools**: Allocate sufficient bandwidth for educational resources, such as video streaming for lectures and large file uploads for assignments and projects.
4. **Accessibility to learning technologies**: Provide equitable access to digital tools and technologies necessary for varied learning activities, ensuring all students have the resources needed to participate fully in digital learning.
5. **Ongoing technological updates**: Regularly update digital learning platforms and tools to incorporate advanced features that enhance educational experiences, such as virtual labs or augmented reality.

8.3.4 Development and Training of Your Team

You will need to invest in faculty and educator development programs to equip your faculty with the necessary skills and knowledge to effectively use digital tools and technologies in teaching and learning. Providing ongoing training and support will help your team adapt to the ever-changing digital learning landscape.

(Further details on the specialised skill sets required to design, develop, and implement online education are discussed in Chap. 2.)

1. **Needs assessment**: Begin with a thorough analysis of the current digital skill levels among faculty. This could involve surveys, interviews, or reviews of past technology use in teaching. The goal is to pinpoint areas where training is most needed.
2. **Customised training programs**: Create targeted training programs that address the identified needs. These could range from basic digital literacy to advanced instructional design. Offer various formats, such as online courses, in-person workshops, or hybrid models.
3. **Peer-led workshops**: Set up opportunities for faculty to learn from colleagues who have successfully integrated digital tools into their teaching. This peer-led approach promotes the sharing of best practices within the community.
4. **Ongoing support structures**: Establish a dedicated team or helpdesk to provide continuous support to faculty as they implement digital tools. This could include technical support, pedagogical consulting, and troubleshooting.
5. **Incentivise participation**: Motivate faculty to participate in development programs by recognizing their efforts, perhaps through certifications, stipends, or acknowledgments in their professional development records.
6. **Evaluate and revise programs**: Implement a feedback loop to assess the impact of the training programs. Use faculty feedback and student outcomes to make data-driven improvements to the programs.
7. **Promote a culture of continuous learning**: Cultivate an environment that encourages faculty to regularly update their skills and knowledge. This could be supported by institutional policies that prioritize and reward ongoing professional development.

8.3.4.1 Case Study: Specialist Postgraduate Medical College

A specialist postgraduate medical college recently enhanced the digital competencies of its teaching faculty by investing in comprehensive development programs. They began with a thorough analysis of current digital skill levels through surveys, interviews, and reviews of past technology use. This assessment highlighted significant variations in digital literacy, identifying areas where training was most needed.

The college then created targeted training programs to address these gaps, ranging from basic digital literacy to advanced instructional design. These programs were offered in various formats, including online courses, in-person workshops, and hybrid models, ensuring accessibility for all faculty members. Peer-led workshops were organised, allowing faculty who had successfully integrated digital tools to share best practices, fostering a supportive community.

To ensure sustained adoption of the tools, the college established a dedicated helpdesk and support team. This team provided technical support, pedagogical consulting, and troubleshooting assistance. To motivate participation, the college offered incentives such as certifications, stipends, and professional development acknowledgments.

The college implemented a feedback loop to assess the training programs' impact, gathering input from faculty and students to make data-driven improvements. Institutional policies prioritised and rewarded ongoing professional development, encouraging faculty to regularly update their skills and knowledge.

By addressing specific needs, providing continuous support, and promoting a culture of continuous learning, the college successfully integrated digital tools into teaching practices, navigating the challenges of the digital learning landscape.

8.3.5 Assessment and Evaluation

Universities should establish effective methods for assessing and evaluating the impact of digital learning initiatives. This includes measuring student outcomes, collecting feedback from stakeholders, and continuously refining the digital learning strategies based on the results.

1. **Develop Key Performance Indicators (KPIs)**: Define clear and measurable KPIs such as course completion rates, grades, and student engagement metrics. These should be aligned with the learning objectives and outcomes that the digital initiative aims to achieve.
2. **Gather stakeholder feedback**: Regularly collect feedback through structured surveys, informal feedback sessions, and discussion forums. This should capture the experiences and satisfaction levels of students, faculty, and staff with the digital learning environment.
3. **Data analysis**: Leverage learning analytics to track and analyse student interaction data from the learning management system (LMS). Use this data to uncover patterns and insights related to student learning behaviours and outcomes.
4. **Continuous refinement**: Create a process for periodic review of digital learning initiatives using the collected data and feedback. Use this information to refine and enhance the learning strategies, tools, and content.
5. **Reporting mechanisms**: Develop transparent reporting mechanisms to communicate the findings from the data analysis to all stakeholders. Ensure that the reports are clear, actionable, and lead to continuous improvement of the digital learning process.

8.3.5.1 Case Study: Assessment and Evaluation in a Medical Faculty

A medical faculty at a prominent university embarked on a digital learning initiative aimed at enhancing educational outcomes and improving student engagement. The faculty faced a particular challenge: integrating digital tools into highly technical, hands-on anatomy courses. To tackle this, they implemented a structured approach to assess and evaluate the impact of their digital learning initiatives.

Strengths of the Approach:

- **Clear KPI Development:** The faculty developed Key Performance Indicators (KPIs) that were aligned with learning objectives, including metrics such as course completion rates, grades, and student engagement. This provided a solid foundation for tracking progress and measuring the effectiveness of digital learning interventions.
- **Stakeholder Feedback:** They actively gathered feedback from students, faculty, and staff through structured surveys, informal feedback sessions, and discussion forums. This open feedback loop helped identify pain points and areas for improvement early in the process.
- **Leveraging Learning Analytics:** By analysing student interaction data from the Learning Management System (LMS), the faculty gained valuable insights into learning behaviours and engagement levels. This data-driven approach allowed for evidence-based decision-making, enabling continuous adjustments to the digital tools.
- **Innovative Solutions:** To address challenges in courses requiring hands-on laboratory work, the faculty introduced virtual labs and simulations. These tools provided students with alternative ways to engage with practical components, even in a digital format.

Weaknesses of the Approach:

- **Limited Adaptation for Practical Courses:** Despite the introduction of virtual labs, some hands-on courses still struggled to fully replicate the in-person experience. Students and faculty reported difficulties in mastering certain technical skills that required physical manipulation of tools or equipment.
- **Inconsistent Faculty Buy-In:** While some faculty members quickly embraced the digital transformation, others were resistant or required more time to adapt. This inconsistency in faculty readiness created uneven experiences for students across different courses.
- **Over-reliance on Learning Analytics:** While analytics provided valuable insights, there was a tendency to over-rely on quantitative data. This sometimes-overlooked qualitative aspects of the learning experience, such as student well-being or the depth of understanding in complex topics.

The medical faculty's approach to digital transformation showcased several commendable practices, particularly in their proactive use of data and continuous refinement of strategies. By collecting both quantitative data through learning analytics and qualitative feedback from stakeholders, they were able to adjust and improve their digital tools in real-time, demonstrating adaptability. However, despite these strengths, challenges remained, particularly in replicating hands-on learning experiences and ensuring consistent faculty buy-in. To improve, the faculty could enhance support for practical courses through technologies like augmented reality, and provide more targeted, phased training for reluctant faculty members. Additionally, balancing the reliance on learning analytics with more nuanced, qualitative insights would offer a comprehensive view of both student performance and satisfaction.

To further enhance their digital learning initiative, the faculty could focus on several key areas for improvement. First, investing in advanced technologies such as augmented or virtual reality could better simulate the hands-on experiences required for technical courses, bridging the gap between theoretical and practical learning. Second, faculty development programs should be more personalized, offering targeted support to those who are resistant or slower to adopt digital tools. Peer mentoring or phased onboarding could help ease these transitions. Finally, while learning analytics provided valuable insights, a more balanced approach that includes qualitative feedback from students and faculty, such as through interviews or focus groups, would offer a more holistic understanding of the learning experience, ensuring both performance metrics and deeper learning needs are met.

8.4 Tips and Tricks

As discussed in the planning section above, risk assessment is a critical part of the digital transformation process. Working through the steps in the following Digital Transformation Risk Assessment Tool [6] helps identify and assess risks across six key areas, evaluate their likely impact, determine mitigation strategies and track and report on these risks.

8.4.1 Digital Transformation Risk Assessment Tool

8.4.1.1 Risk Identification

The first step involves identifying potential risks across different areas of the transformation. This can be categorised into:

- **Technical Risks**: Issues related to infrastructure, software, and hardware failure.
- **Human Resources Risks**: Faculty resistance, lack of skills, or insufficient training.
- **Operational Risks**: Disruptions in service delivery, poor student experience, and data security.
- **Financial Risks**: Budget overruns, unforeseen costs, or inadequate resource allocation.

Table 8.2 Risk Evaluation Matrix

Risk	Likelihood (Low, Medium, High)	Impact (Low, Medium, High)	Priority (Low, Medium, High)
Technical failure	High	High	High
Faculty resistance	Medium	High	Medium
Budget overrun	Low	Medium	Low
Data privacy non-compliance	Low	High	Medium
Student dissatisfaction	Medium	High	High

- **Regulatory Risks**: Non-compliance with data privacy laws or accreditation standards.
- **Reputation Risks**: Negative feedback from stakeholders, damaging public image.

8.4.1.2 Risk Evaluation Matrix

Each risk identified is evaluated using a two-dimensional matrix with "Likelihood" and "Impact" scales. This allows prioritization of risks (See Table 8.2).

8.4.1.3 Mitigation Strategies

For each risk, a corresponding mitigation strategy is identified to reduce likelihood or impact (See Table 8.3).

8.4.1.4 Monitoring and Reporting

Establish monitoring mechanisms to track risks over time. Use a risk dashboard to continuously assess risk exposure (See Table 8.4).

8.4.1.5 Contingency Planning

Develop contingency plans for high-priority risks. These should include:
- **Action Plan**: Steps to take if the risk materializes.
- **Resources Required**: Budget, staff, or technological resources needed to manage the risk.
- **Responsible Person(s)**: Individual(s) assigned to manage the contingency.

Table 8.3 Mitigation Strategies

Risk	Mitigation strategy
Technical failure	Ensure redundancy in systems, backup critical data, perform regular system maintenance.
Faculty resistance	Provide personalized, ongoing training and support, include faculty in decision-making.
Budget overrun	Develop a detailed project budget with contingency funds, track expenses closely.
Data privacy non-compliance	Ensure compliance with data privacy regulations like, FERPA (The Family Educational Rights and Privacy Act), HIPAA (The Health Insurance Portability and Accountability Act), GDPR (General Data Protection Regulation), provide security training.
Student dissatisfaction	Collect regular feedback, improve engagement through enhanced communication.

Table 8.4 Monitoring and Reporting

Risk	Current status	Action taken	Next steps
Technical failure	Under control	Implemented system backups	Review new technological solutions
Faculty resistance	Rising	Launched additional workshops	Schedule peer mentoring sessions
Budget overrun	Stable	Reallocated contingency funds	Continue close tracking
Data privacy non-compliance	Low	Privacy policies reviewed	Ongoing staff training in data protection
Student dissatisfaction	Moderate	Surveys conducted and analysed	Implement changes in online course design

8.5 Conclusion

Leading and implementing a digital learning transformation is a thrilling opportunity to shape the future of education. As leaders, you have the power to drive this change by embracing the potential of technology, fostering a culture of innovation, and supporting your faculty and students throughout the journey. By investing in robust infrastructure, providing comprehensive training, and continuously ensuring quality, you can overcome resistance and create a dynamic, inclusive, and forward-thinking educational environment. Remember, your leadership will not only enhance learning experiences but also equip students with the skills they need for a rapidly evolving world. Take the reins, inspire your team, and lead the way in transforming learning for the better.

References

1. Liu Q, Geertshuis S, Grainger R. Understanding academics' adoption of learning technologies: a systematic review. Comput Educ [Internet]. 2020 Jul 1 [cited 2024 Nov 22];151:103857. Available from: https://research.ebsco.com/linkprocessor/plink?id=bbd027b8-3f5e-3f71-ab6a-8321fc87ffbc
2. Velthuis F, Varpio L, Helmich E, Dekker H, Jaarsma ADC. Navigating the complexities of undergraduate medical curriculum change: change leaders' perspectives. Acad Med [Internet]. 2018 Oct 1 [cited 2024 Nov 22];93(10):1503–10. Available from: https://research.ebsco.com/linkprocessor/plink?id=d2616632-a658-33b7-a82a-22497d6dc5f5
3. Porter WW, Graham CR. Institutional drivers and barriers to faculty adoption of blended learning in higher education. Br J Educ Technol [Internet]. 2016 Jul 1 [cited 2024 Nov 22];47(4):748–62. Available from: https://research.ebsco.com/linkprocessor/plink?id=7b400aa3-a88d-34e7-b2f9-09ef1831e38d
4. King E, Boyatt R. Exploring factors that influence adoption of e-learning within higher education. Br J Educ Technol [Internet]. 2015 Nov 1 [cited 2024 Nov 22];46(6):1272–80. Available from: https://research.ebsco.com/linkprocessor/plink?id=6b125fcd-21d9-3e98-b6fe-b5a04c4b8c76
5. Li Y, Lindner JR. Faculty adoption behaviour about web-based distance education: a case study from China Agricultural University. Br J Educ Technol [Internet]. 2007 Jan 1 [cited 2024 Nov 22];38(1):83–94. Available from: https://research.ebsco.com/linkprocessor/plink?id=42b5c04a-c6eb-3d61-9ecd-2a02d0185a36
6. Bowser D. Digital transformation risk assessment tool [cited 2024 Nov 22].

Made in the USA
Monee, IL
03 May 2026

49438635R00122